Preparing for a Healthy Baby

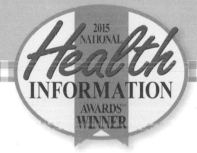

Preparing For A Healthy Baby – 2014 Edition

This book is intended as an informational guide. In no way is this book intended to replace, countermand, or conflict with the advice given to you by your OB provider. This author and Trimester, Inc. take no responsibility for any consequences from any course of action suggested in this book. **Always call your OB provider with questions.**

Copyright © 2014 Trimester, Inc.

All rights reserved. No part of this publication may be reproduced, stored in a retrieval system or transmitted, in any form or by many means, electronic, mechanical, photocopying, recording or otherwise, without prior written permission of Trimester, Inc. Printed in the United States of America.

Published by Trimester, Inc.
www.HealthyBabyBook.com

Trimester, Inc, edition February 2014
ISBN: 978-0-9789275-0-9 *English*
ISBN: 978-0-978975-1-6 *Spanish*

Preparing For A Healthy Baby is available at special discounts for bulk purchases in the U.S. by doctor offices, corporations, institutions, and other organizations.

For more information visit www.HealthyBabyBook.com or contact Trimester, Inc. at (800) 841-5205, orders@healthybabybook.com or fax (602) 840-9685.

Single copies of this book may be purchased on our website www.HealthyBabyBook.com or on Amazon.com.

Table of Contents

Introduction

Congratulations!

You are about to experience the universal and normal process of having a baby. You probably have many questions about how to provide the best possible care for the newest member of your family.

All of these questions and many more will be answered in this book.

- What body changes can you expect?
- What foods are best to eat while you are pregnant?
- Which substances are potentially dangerous to you and your new baby?
- What exercises are helpful during pregnancy?
- How is the baby growing month-by-month?
- What will occur during regular office appointments?
- What can you expect during labor and delivery?

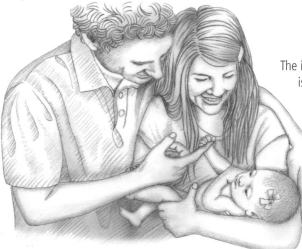

The information in this book is meant to be used as a supplement to your prenatal education and care. This book cannot be used by itself without the expert guidance of your OB provider. It is important to remember every woman is different and so is every pregnancy.

In order for you to keep track of your appointments and your progress, an "Appointment Record" is included at the beginning of this book. Ask your OB provider to keep it updated for you and make a note for your next appointment so it will be easier to remember. There are several blank pages throughout this book. Please use these pages to note questions you may wish to ask at your prenatal classes and during appointments. This book has been designed to be small enough to fit into most purses for easy transport back and forth to your classes and OB provider's office.

Keeping Healthy During Pregnancy

Importance of Early Regular Medical Visits

First Visit to the OB Office

History
During your first visit to the OB office, a medical, family and pregnancy history is usually obtained. From this information, your OB provider will be able to give you some idea if there are any problems in these areas that should be considered during your pregnancy.

Physical
An obstetrical physical and pelvic exam is also usually done. This informs the OB provider of any physical problems that might affect your pregnancy.

Lab Tests
Various blood tests and cultures are usually done to obtain information needed to monitor you and your baby's health. A list of these are included in this book under the heading "Prenatal Testing." Ask your provider to fill out your blood type on your "Appointment Record".

Delivery Date
On the initial visit, your "due date" will be calculated. Your "due date" is just an estimate. A baby may be born before or as much as two weeks after this date. The most common method used to calculate your "due date" is to count back three months from the first day of the last menstrual period (LMP) and add seven days.
This time period is 280 days or forty weeks.

Drugs, Alcohol, Smoking, and Chemical Exposure
The use of drugs and alcohol, smoking, and exposure to chemicals found in the home or workplaces are subjects usually discussed early in your pregnancy. Most providers prefer you take no medications in the first 12 weeks (3 months) of your pregnancy. After this time, medications ("over-the-counter" or prescription) should be taken on the advice of your OB provider. The use of alcohol as well as smoking can damage the baby. Please discuss this with your OB provider during your initial visit. Your work and home environment should also be discussed to determine if there could be possible exposure to any chemicals there that could damage the baby.

Appointment Record

Routine Visits to Your OB Office

Visits after the initial one may seem short, but they are very important. Each time you will have your weight, urine and blood pressure checked. The baby's growth and heartbeat will be evaluated. By checking these things and listening to any questions you have, or problems you may be experiencing and are concerned about, it will be possible for your OB provider to detect early problems that may affect you and your baby. If all is going well, you will probably be seen every 4-6 weeks for the first six months, every 2-3 weeks in your seventh and eighth month and every 1-2 weeks in your last month.

My OB Provider's Name: _____

My OB Provider's Phone #: _____ Hospital: _____

Due Date: _____ Blood Type & Rh: _____

Date	Weight	Blood Pressure	Urine	Other

Emotional Changes During Pregnancy

Pregnancy is a time of change for a woman's body, in order to meet the needs of the growing baby. There are many common and predictable changes, yet each woman experiences each of her pregnancies differently.

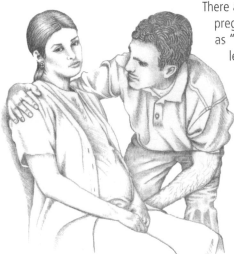

There are many emotional changes that occur in pregnancy. Many times these are referred to as "mood swings." The increasing hormone level can cause you to be tearful one moment and laughing the next. You may notice a decrease in sexual interest, but the opposite may also be true. Your partner may also have new feelings, concerns, and worries about himself or about you, your relationship with him, and your changing body. The responsibilities of raising a child may be scary or exciting. Pregnancy can bring many changes into your life.

Emotional confusion and mood swings are normal.

Be sure to jot down any concerns and feel free to bring them up with your partner and/or your OB provider. Usually during the mid-pregnancy period, you will find yourself less tired and many of the early discomforts of pregnancy disappear. You and your partner will feel better, both physically and emotionally.

As you come into the last three months of pregnancy, you will find labor and delivery occupying your thoughts. You may find that the things your relatives, co-workers and friends tell you may cause concern. Be sure to discuss these concerns or any fears you have with your OB provider. Prepared Childbirth Classes will eliminate many of these fears and help you manage your own body during labor and delivery.

Weight Gain During Pregnancy

Gaining Weight

Gaining weight is healthy during pregnancy to allow for the body changes that occur. When you gain your weight and how much you gain is important for a healthy baby. To help you look at the pattern of your weight gain, a chart is provided for you to plot your weight gain throughout the course of your pregnancy. A slow and steady weight gain - about 2 to 4 pounds total during the first 3 months is recommended. After that, a gain of about 3/4 to one pound per week for a total of 24 to 35 pounds, for a woman of average weight prior to pregnancy, is recommended.

Losing Weight

A weight reduction diet while you are pregnant may be unhealthy for you and your baby. Pregnancy is not the time to lose weight. You can lose weight after the baby is born. Check with your OB provider regarding a moderate exercise program. This is a good way to help you control your weight gain.

Eating Properly

"Eating for two" is an old-fashioned concept that has proven to be wrong. Pregnant women need only an additional 300 calories per day for the baby. However, it is important to eat regular meals plus nutritious snacks, as the baby is growing 24 hours a day and needs a steady supply of nutrients and oxygen. Do not skip a meal. If you are gaining too much weight and gaining it too quickly, it may be because you are eating too much and/or eating empty calorie foods high in fat and sugar.

Vitamins and Minerals

By eating a diet of the correct serving sizes required, you will be receiving most of the nutrients you need for a healthy pregnancy. Additionally, since pregnancy places an increased demand on your body for certain nutrients, your OB provider may recommend a vitamin-mineral supplement. These vitamins should be rich in the B vitamin known as folic acid. (See page 12.)

The following chart is one that shows the average weight gain during pregnancy. You can chart your own weight gain here and see how you compare.

Average Weight Gain

1½	lbs.	Placenta
2	lbs.	Uterus
2	lbs.	Breast tissue increase
8½	lbs.	Increased blood/fluids
7½	lbs.	Baby
7	lbs.	Extra fat/tissue (necessary)
28+	**lbs.**	**Total Weight Gain**

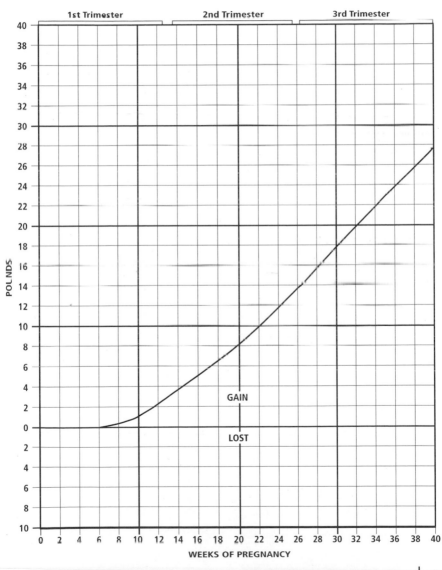

Nutrition During Pregnancy

What can and should I eat?

It is important to eat food that will keep you healthy. A balanced diet gives you what you need for the changes in your body. Good food also helps your baby grow and develop. A healthy baby has fewer problems. Avoid high-calorie, high-fat and low-nutrient foods such as candy, soft drinks and high-fat, sugary snack foods. They add calories and give few of the vitamins and minerals that you need. Only 30% of daily calories should be from fats. Try to limit the use of butter, gravy and heavy dressing. Deserts and sugary soft drinks should only be a special treat. You may use salt unless your health advisor tells you otherwise.

You should obtain prenatal vitamins from the pharmacy and take one daily. These are not meant as a replacement for good nutrition but are only a supplement. Do not take any vitamins without checking with your OB provider. Follow the daily food guide below. It will help you choose your servings from each food group. You should also follow the guide if you breast-feed your baby.

Water and other Liquids: Drink 6 to 8 glasses every day. This includes fruit juices, soups and other beverages. Liquids help in many ways:

- They help the blood circulate.
- They help the body fluids circulate.
- They help the digestion of food.
- They can help prevent constipation.
- They can prevent urinary tract infections.

Food Group / Function

Grain Group (Whole Grain/Enriched)
- Good source of Vitamin B-1 which makes energy available from food eaten.
- Iron helps make hemoglobin, the red substance in blood that carries oxygen to the cells.

Note: Try to eat ½ of your daily grains that are 100% whole grain

Daily Food Guide

Minimum Servings per Day: 6 ounces

Bread	1 slice
Rolls, buns.	1 of either
Tortilla (corn or flour)	1 (6-inch)
Cereal, rice, macaroni, spaghetti, cooked	½ cup
Cereal, ready to eat.	1 cup
Crackers.	1 ounce or 5

Food Group / Function

Daily Food Guide

Vegetable Group
- Helps develop your baby's skeleton, eyes, skin, hair, teeth, gums and glands.
- Keep your skin and hair healthy.
- Helps develop good vision.

Note: Wash all vegetables thoroughly with water.

Minimum Servings per Day: 2½ cups

Spinach, collards, kale, mustard greens, bok choy, swiss chard . . . . 2 cups

Deep green lettuce . . . . 2 cups
(red leaf, romaine, and endive)

Carrots, winter squash, sweet potatoes, apricots . . . . ½ cup

Green beans, peas, pears, celery, beets, grapes . . . . ½ cup

Fruit Group
- Forms healthy bones, teeth and gums.
- Builds strong body cells.
- Helps in healing wounds.
- Helps the body use iron

Note: Wash all fruits thoroughly with water.

Minimum Servings per Day: 1½ -2 cups

1 cup is equal to:

Apple . . . 1 small or 1 cup sliced/chopped

Applesauce . . . . 1 cup

Dried fruit . . . . 1/2 cup

Orange, grapefruit, banana . . . . . . 1 small

Orange, grapefruit juice . . . . 1 cup

Grapes . . . . 1 cup

Dairy Group
- Helps build strong bones and teeth.
- Helps nerves and muscles react normally.
- Has many vitamins, proteins and minerals.

Note: All milk products should be pasteurized. Try to use fat-free or low-fat dairy products

Minimum Servings per Day: 3 cups

Milk . . . . 1 cup
all kinds, including non-fat dry milk, buttermilk

Cheese . . . . 1½ ounces

Cottage cheese . . . . 2 cups

Ice cream (fat-free or low fat) . . . 1½ cups

Yogurt . . . . 1 cup

Protein Group
Protein is the basic building material for you and your baby.
- It helps your baby grow.
- It builds and repairs tissues.
- It forms antibodies that fight infection.
- It helps build blood and supplies energy.

Note: Have at least 1 serving from vegetable protein. Avoid raw/uncooked meat, poultry, eggs, or fish. Choose lean meat and poultry.

Minimum Servings per Day: 5-6
Animal Protein:

Cooked lean meat, fish, poultry . . 1 ounce

Egg . . . . 1 large

Luncheon meat . . . . 1 slice

Vegetable Protein:

Cooked, dried beans, peas, lentils . . ¼ cup

Tofu . . . . 2 ounces or ¼ cup

Peanuts, pumpkin or sunflower seeds . . . . ½ ounce or ⅛ cup

Almonds, walnuts or pistachios . . ½ ounce

Hummus . . . . 2 Tbsp.

Peanut butter . . . . 1 Tbsp.

Snack Foods

Snack foods should not be "junk food." Junk food is described as any food that contains few or no nutrients for each calorie. These are usually foods that are too high in sugar/fat/salt or artificial ingredients. In pregnancy, you and your baby need many nutrients to be healthy. Empty calories provide few nutrients and contribute to fat weight instead of the proper weight gain of lean tissue. Replace any junk foods you are eating with similar foods that are high in nutrients. Remember, some of these substitutes may be high in calories.

Healthy Snack Foods:
- Whole grain crackers - wheat, rye, corn, or rice.
- Popcorn (no butter).
- Dry cereals - read the label to see that little or no sugar and fats are added.
- Fresh fruits such as apples or citrus.
- Pretzels (unsalted) - have less fat than potato chips.
- Fresh vegetables - carrots, celery, radishes, zucchini, mushrooms, tomatoes, green peppers.
- Nuts or seeds (in the shell) - having to shell them keeps a person from eating too many, too fast. If you are watching the fats in your diet, you may want to avoid these.
- Dips made with plain yogurt or cottage cheese, instead of mayonnaise or sour cream. Use raw vegetables to dip with!
- Cheese, with crackers or fruit.

Fast Foods:
(Including hamburgers, fried chicken, pizza, french fries, shakes, tacos)
Generally, these foods do have some nutrients and protein, but they can be too high in fat, sugar and salt. Often fast food meals don't have sufficient servings of fruit and vegetables. Continue to enjoy eating out, but limit your fast food meals to once a week if gaining too much weight is a problem for you. Also, on those days you eat fast foods, include more servings of fruits and vegetables in your other meals. Salad bars are good, but watch the amount of dressing you use. Look for restaurants or cafeterias where a variety of lean meat, fish, fruits, and vegetables are available.

Instead of Candy:

- Try dried fruit – apples, dates, raisins, prunes, pineapple, apricots, peaches.

- Try ice-cold fresh fruit or juices.

- Try frozen unsweetened fruit – Bing cherries, strawberries, peaches, grapes, bananas or melon balls. Eat before completely thawed.

- Try fruit canned in its own juice.

- Try fruit combinations – apples with peanut butter, pears with cheese.

Instead of cakes, pies, cookies, donuts, sweet rolls:

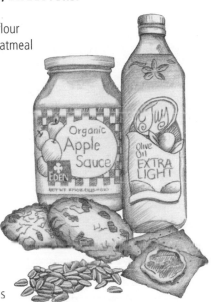

- Make your own cookies with nutritious ingredients, such as: substitute whole wheat flour for white flour; choose applesauce, raisin or oatmeal cookie recipes; add raisins, nuts, or chopped dried fruit in place of chocolate chips.

- Try using less fat and sugar in your cooking and baking. For each cup of shortening or sugar, use 2 tablespoons less than the recipe calls for. Try substituting polyunsaturated oil (safflower, corn, soybean), margarine with extra light olive oil. When baking, try using applesauce instead of oil in your recipes.

- Try rice or bread pudding; ice milk; pudding or custard made with lowfat milk; whole grain crackers spread with peanut butter.

- Mix ¾ cup lowfat yogurt with 2 tablespoons orange juice concentrate; eat as is or freeze as popsicles.

Salt:

Sodium (salt) is a necessary mineral element for the health of the pregnant woman. If your OB provider requests that you limit salt, it can be done in the following manner:

- Light use of salt in cooking, but none added at the table.

- No obviously salty foods (such as canned vegetables, canned soup, ham, hot dogs, lunchmeats, bacon, potato chips, salted nuts) or salty condiments (pickles, olives, salad dressings, catsup).

There are a variety of herbs and spices to enhance the flavor of foods as a substitute for salt: thyme, onion, garlic, parsley, rosemary, oregano, mushrooms, chives, ginger, and lemon to name a few.

Calcium:

In addition to your calcium needs, calcium is essential in building your baby's bones and teeth. If you do not eat or drink enough calcium, your baby will take calcium from your bones. This can lead to osteoporosis (fragile bones) and loss of your teeth. Pregnant women should get 1,000 to 1,300 mg of calcium each day. If you don't like milk, you can substitute the following:

1 cup milk	=	1 cup yogurt (low fat)
⅔ cup milk	=	1 slice (1 oz.) cheddar cheese (low fat may be used)
⅔ cup milk	=	3 oz. canned salmon including bones
¼ cup milk	=	½ cup cottage cheese (low fat may be used)
½ cup milk	=	½ cup custard/milk pudding (low fat may be used)

Other foods that are a good source of calcium:
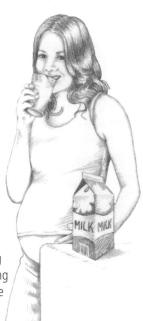
- Dark green vegetables (collard, kale, turnip, mustard and spinach greens)
- Fortified orange juice
- Sardines
- Nuts and seeds

If you are unable to tolerate these foods or cannot take at least 3 servings a day, consult your OB provider for a calcium supplement.

Folic Acid:

This B vitamin helps prevent certain spinal and brain defects that could form in the baby. If a woman thinks she may become pregnant or already is pregnant, this vitamin should be taken every day. The recommended intake is .4mg (400 micrograms) of folic acid every day. NOT more than 1mg or 1000 micrograms should be taken unless your health care provider recommends it.

Foods High in Folic Acid (folate) - 80mcg or mor
Asparagus, breakfast cereals, Brewer's yeast, garbanzo beans, lentils, liver, mustard greens, orange juice, spinach, strawberries and sunflower seeds.

Foods Moderately High in Folic Acid (folate) - 40 - 80mcg
Artichokes, avocados, beets, broccoli, brussel sprouts, cantaloupe, cauliflower, corn, green peas, okra, oranges, papayas, peanuts, raspberries, salad greens, split peas and wheat germ.

High Iron Foods

Your hemoglobin and hematocrit, which are measures of the amount of iron in your blood, may be lower during pregnancy. It is important that you increase your intake of iron. You can do this by including more of the following foods in your diet. The recommended dietary allowance (RDA) of iron during pregnancy is 30 milligrams (mg). Here are some foods rich in iron. Eat as many foods from these high-iron foods as often as you can.

Foods that provide 3 to 12 mg of Iron

Clams	4 large or 9 small
Oysters	6 medium
Spinach	½ cup cooked
Fortified cereal	1 cup
Dates	1 cup
Dried apricots	17 halves
Black walnuts	½ cup
Peanuts	½ cup
Sunflower seed kernels	4 ounces
Prunes	10 large
Prune juice	1 cup
Cream of Wheat enriched	1 cup

Foods that provide 1.6 to 3 mg of Iron

Sirloin steak	3 ounces
Roast beef	3 ounces
Lean hamburger	3 ounces
Baked potato with skin	1 whole
Kidney beans	½ cup cooked
Lima beans	½ cup cooked
Navy beans	½ cup cooked
Oatmeal	1 cup cooked
Raisins	½ cup

Foods that provide .5 to 1.5 mg of Iron

Chicken	3 ounces
Green peas	½ cup
Tomato juice	6 ounces
Broccoli	½ cup
Brussel sprouts	½ cup cooked
Whole wheat bread	1 slice
Raspberries	1 cup
Strawberries	1 cup

Additional Sources of Iron

- All kinds of liver (except fish)--however, liver should not be eaten more than once a week
- Lean beef, veal, pork or lamb
- Leafy greens, all kinds
- Beets
- Sauerkraut
- Tofu
- Lentils
- Soy bean flour
- Unrefined sugars, such as molasses

Vitamin C helps your body use iron.

Be sure you are getting one fruit or vegetable that contains Vitamin C every day. This will help your body utilize the iron you eat. The Folacin and Vitamin C from greens are more readily absorbed if cooked and eaten with meat, poultry or fish.

Iron Pills

If your iron level is too low (anemia), your OB provider may suggest iron pills. It is not unusual for your stools to become black or for you to become constipated while taking iron pills. To prevent this, you should increase fresh fruits, vegetables, fiber (bran), and liquids in your diet. Your OB provider may suggest a "bulk producing" substance (such as Metamucil) or a stool softener (such as Colace) if your constipation is not relieved by diet alone.

Caffeine Alternatives

Caffeine is a stimulating chemical found in coffee and some soft drinks (such as Pepsi, Dr. Pepper, Mountain Dew, Coca Cola, etc.) A similar chemical is found in tea and chocolate. At this time doctors don't know all of the effects of caffeine on the unborn child. There is a concern that caffeine stimulates the baby's nervous system much more than it does the mother's. Because the baby is small and immature, the caffeine may have a greater effect on its growing parts and may harm delicate tissues. Therefore, it is best to limit caffeine.

Caffeine Content

Coffee (drip)	146 mg/cup	Dr. Pepper	38 mg/12 oz	Sprite	0 mg/12 oz
Coca-Cola	65 mg/12 oz	Diet Dr. Pepper	38 mg/12 oz	Diet 7-Up	0 mg/12 oz
Mountain Dew	52 mg/12 oz	Pepsi	37 mg/12 oz	Diet Sunkist	0 mg/12 oz
Tea (3 min. brew)	52 mg/12 oz	Diet Pepsi	37 mg/12 oz	Fanta Orange	0 mg/12 oz
Sunkist Orange	42 mg/12 oz	7-Up	0 mg/12 oz	Fresca	0 mg/12 oz

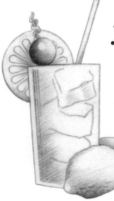

Instead of Caffeine-Containing Drinks, try:
- Decaffeinated coffee.
- Tea that is labeled "no caffeine" in flavors such as peppermint, spearmint, orange, spice or cinnamon.
- Lemonade or any fruit drink you make with real fruit juice.
- Bouillon or broth
- Milk
  - Ice water
    - Soda water with a twist of lime or lemon.
    - For drinks you usually have at one temperature, try them the opposite way, such as hot apple juice with cinnamon, hot lemonade or hot cranberry juice.

Caffeine in Medications:
Some over-the-counter and prescription medications have caffeine added. Read the label and discuss with your OB provider before you take these.

Artificial Sweeteners:
There is no evidence that the use of artificial sweeteners (aspartame and saccharin and others) increases the risk of birth defects. Discuss the use of these with your OB provider.

Alcohol & Drinking Alternatives

When you drink, your unborn baby drinks too. While alcohol may not significantly harm the mother's body, doctors are concerned that a growing baby's delicate tissues may be damaged. Drinking alcohol during pregnancy can result in Fetal Alcohol Syndrome. Fetal Alcohol Syndrome babies are abnormally small at birth, especially in head size, with most of these babies having small brains and some amount of mental retardation that may not improve with age. They have short attention spans and behavioral problems. Some have heart defects, which may require surgery.

The best advice is: Do not drink any beer, wine or liquor while you are pregnant.

Instead of drinking alcoholic beverages:

• Tell people you are not drinking at all while you are pregnant because you are growing one of the world's healthiest, smartest babies.

• When you are away from home, ask for soda water with a lime or a twist of lemon.

• Order fruit juice without the alcohol such as a Screwdriver without vodka, Bloody Mary without vodka (called "Virgin Mary"), or ask for a Shirley Temple, limeade or lemonade made with club soda.

• When you give up drinking, do not use any drugs as a substitute. Take medication only on the advice of your OB provider.

• If you feel the need to drink alcohol when you are pregnant, discuss this with your OB provider.

No Smoking or Using Drugs

Surgeon General's Warning
Smoking by Pregnant Women May Result in Fetal Injury, Premature Birth, and Low Birth Weight.

Cigarettes:
Smoking has been clearly linked to low birth weights (under 51/2 lbs.) and some studies show increased rates of Sudden Infant Death Syndrome (SIDS) also known as crib death. Smoking also increases the risk of miscarriages, stillbirths and premature births. Smoking decreases the amount of oxygen that reaches the placenta, thus depriving the baby of oxygen. There is recent evidence that children of smoking mothers continue to show some growth restriction and learning disabilities. Therefore, women who smoke should not smoke during their pregnancy.

Marijuana:
Smoking marijuana during pregnancy should be avoided. Marijuana has proven to have damaging effects on a number of body systems, similar to cigarettes, and therefore presents risks to the fetus. This drug puts the baby at risk for premature birth, slow fetal growth and withdrawal symptoms.

If you need help to quit smoking, please ask your OB provider for suggestions.

Cocaine:
Babies need food and oxygen to grow. If a pregnant woman uses crack or any form of cocaine, she cuts the food and oxygen supply to the unborn baby causing brain damage or death. Use of cocaine can cause early separation of the placenta from the walls of the uterus, causing the baby to be born early. The baby may even go through withdrawal shortly after birth. This drug can also cause dangerously high blood pressure and heart rate in the mother. If you are pregnant and have already used cocaine, STOP NOW. Discuss this with your OB provider.

Heroin:
This drug puts the pregnant woman at risk for hepatitis, AIDS, and miscarriage. Its use during pregnancy may cause fetal death, slow fetal growth and premature births. Babies are also at greater risk for long term learning disabilities and behavioral problems. The baby may go through withdrawal shortly after birth. Stop the use of this drug immediately and discuss this with your OB provider.

Amphetamines (Methamphetamines):
Use of this drug during pregnancy can cause birth defects in the baby. This drug affects the baby's heart, brain, liver, bones, stomach, kidneys and intestines. These babies may be born at a low birth weight and have ten times greater risk of Sudden Infant Death Syndrome (SIDS) than drug free babies. Learning disabilities may appear as these babies get older. The baby may go through withdrawal symptoms after birth. Stop the use of this drug immediately and discuss this with your OB provider.

Health Alerts

*The flu vaccine is recommended by
the Center for Disease Control (CDC)
for all pregnant women*

The following are considerations to keep in mind during pregnancy.

Aerosols, Insecticides, and Paint

Anything that is an organic chemical base may enter the bloodstream and may be passed on to the baby. Avoid using these things while you are pregnant. If you must use these materials, have good ventilation and avoid breathing the vapors. Use a mask.

Cats, Raw Meat

Cats are the primary carriers of "toxoplasmosis," an infection that can cause birth defects. This organism is found in the raw meat and the feces of cats. To avoid this disease, wash your hands after handling cats, don't empty kitty litter, and don't eat raw meat. When gardening use gloves; cats may use your garden as a litter box.

Colds or Flu

- Check your temperature twice a day. If over 100.3°F, call your doctor.
- Increase your fluids (10 to 12 glasses per day).
- Maintain balanced nutrition.
- Increase your rest.
- Use a cool-mist humidifier when sleeping.

Call your OB provider if:

- your temperature is over 100.3°F.
- your chest hurts, you are coughing up green mucous or you are short of breath.
- you have a severe sore throat and are having trouble swallowing.
- your cough, congestion or sore throat continues for more than 7-10 days.
- you feel that you may need to use a medication, prescription or over-the-counter drug.

Dental Work

Your mouth's bacteria and acid/alkaline balance change during pregnancy, and this may make you more prone to cavities. It is a good idea to have a professional cleaning of teeth and gums early in pregnancy to prevent inflammation of gums that many women experience. Inform your dentist that you are pregnant. X-rays should be avoided. If necessary, dental x-rays may be taken later in pregnancy if a protective lead shield is used. It is better to wait until after the baby is born for any elective dental work or x-rays.

Diarrhea

Diarrhea is the frequent passage of watery bowel movements. If you develop diarrhea, do the following:

- Check for uterine contractions (see "Preterm Labor," page 48).
- Drink clear liquids for 24 hours (tea, Jell-o, Gatorade, Sprite, 7-Up, popsicles or broth).
- Avoid or limit fruit juices.
- Eat bland foods for the next 24 to 48 hours (cottage cheese, cheese, plain yogurt, bananas, applesauce, baked potatoes, crackers or plain toast, white rice).
- Increase your foods slowly to your normal routine.
- If the above doesn't help, call your OB provider.
- If there are more than 6 bowel movements in a day, or other symptoms, call your OB provider to discuss possible medication. Do not use Pepto Bismol for diarrhea because it contains aspirin.

Douching

There is usually no need to douche while you are pregnant. Air could be introduced into your circulatory system from the pressure of the solution and cause problems for you and your pregnancy.

Immunizations

Vaccines can protect you and your baby against some potentially serious infections. Some vaccines are safe in pregnancy, and others are not. Your provider can tell you what vaccines are right for you during and after pregnancy.

- **Flu vaccines:** Pregnant women who come down with the flu are more likely than other adults to have serious complication, such as pneumonia. The flu vaccination protects the mother as well as the baby. Babies should not get vaccinated against the flu until they are about six months old, but they will receive protection from their mother that received the flu vaccination until they can be vaccinated. The U.S. Center for Disease Control and Prevention (CDC) encourage all pregnant and postpartum women to get the seasonal flu vaccine. This shot is made from killed viruses and is safe for mother and baby. Family members may also want to consider getting the flu shot.

- **Hepatitis B vaccines:** If you are at risk for Hepatitis B (work in a health care facility, travel to areas of infection or have certain chronic health conditions), you should talk to your provider about receiving this vaccination. The Hepatitis B vaccine does not contain live viruses and limited studies show there are no apparent risks for the developing baby.

- **Vaccines to avoid:** According to the CDC the following live-virus vaccines are not recommended during pregnancy: nasal spray flu vaccines (flu shot are recommended), measles, mumps, rubella (German measles), chickenpox (varicella) and tuberculosis (BCG). The human papillomavirus (HPV) appears to be safe for both mother and baby but it is still being studied and has not been approved for use during pregnancy. Other vaccination or immunizations should be discussed with your provider.

Medications
Pregnant women should avoid taking any medication, prescription or over-the-counter. Consult with your OB provider before taking any medications.

Rubella
Also known as the "three-day measles" or "German measles," this is a communicable virus that usually occurs before adolescence. An episode of pre-pregnancy measles usually gives immunity to the individual. A blood test is done early in pregnancy to determine if you have immunity to Rubella.

The first symptom noticed is a rash that starts on the face and spreads to the body, arms and legs. Headache, sore throat, and loss of appetite may also occur.

If a pregnant woman gets Rubella, it can create problems for the fetus. Rubella in the first 3 months of pregnancy can lead to a miscarriage or to fetal defects.

It is important for pregnant women who have no immunity to Rubella to avoid contact with people who have an active case. After delivery, a woman with no immunity to Rubella should be immunized.

Saunas, Hot Tubs
The uses of these are not recommended in pregnancy. The extreme temperatures could potentially damage the developing baby. Do not take extremely hot baths; temperatures should be below 100°F.

Seafood
The U.S. Food and Drug Administration has advised pregnant women to avoid consuming large amounts of fish, including swordfish, shark, king mackerel and tilefish. These fish may have accumulated unsafe levels of mercury from the ocean. A moderate amount (12 ounces or less per week) of other fish, such as tuna, is probably safe during pregnancy. Albacore (white) tuna has more mercury than canned light tuna. Albacore tuna should be eaten only up to 6 ounces each week. Local health departments should be contacted for additional information on the fish caught and sold in each local area. Fish oil capsules may be taken as directed by your OB provider.

Work
Pregnant women can work up to delivery in most cases. Individual restrictions will be evaluated by your OB provider based on the needs of your pregnancy.

X-Rays
Avoid contact if possible. It is best to avoid x-rays, including dental x-rays, during pregnancy. Consult with your OB provider if they are indicated. Women should request an x-ray shield with any x-ray.

Sexually Transmitted Diseases

Chlamydia

Chlamydia is one of the most common sexually transmitted diseases in the United States today. Many women have few or no symptoms. Those who do have symptoms may get them anywhere from 2 days to 3 weeks after sexual contact with a person who has the disease. Chlamydia is an organism that commonly infects the cervix and may spread to the uterus and fallopian tubes. Chlamydia infections can lead to infertility problems (difficulty getting pregnant) or ectopic or tubal pregnancies. Symptoms include: a yellowish vaginal discharge, pain or burning during urination, burning or itching in the genital area and pain with intercourse. A pregnant woman with Chlamydia can transmit the disease to her infant during birth. The most frequent result is an eye infection that is easily treated. But there are more serious problems, such as pneumonia, that may require hospitalization. Pre-term labor is also more common in pregnant women with Chlamydia. Early detection and treatment of this disease are very important to assist in having a healthy baby.

Genital Herpes or HSV (Herpes Simplex Virus)

Genital herpes is a sexually transmitted viral disease that may show symptoms from 2 to 20 days after contact. Females will have a blister or a group of blisters in the genital area that may cause discomfort or pain. The virus can remain dormant for long periods of time with no other outbreaks. Some women may have frequent outbreaks of the blisters. Regardless of your symptoms, any history of genital herpes in yourself or partner should be reported to your OB provider. During pregnancy, sexual relations should be avoided when blisters are present or suspected on self or partner. It is important to inform your OB provider of any outbreaks during your pregnancy. Your provider may choose to use a medication to shorten the time of these outbreaks. A positive culture or active blister prior to delivery may indicate the need for a Cesarean delivery to prevent infection to the infant.

Genital warts (Condylomata)

Genital warts are caused by a virus called human papillomavirus (HPV). This virus is sexually transmitted. Genital warts can grow very quickly when you are pregnant. In rare cases, they can even block the birth canal. Your condition will need to be followed closely by your OB provider during your pregnancy. After delivery, it is important to have regular pap smears. This virus can go up inside the uterus and possibly infect the cervix, that can result in cervical cancer.

Gonorrhea

Gonorrhea is a common sexually transmitted disease. Many women have no symptoms. Therefore, any sexual contact with a partner thought to be infected should be reported to your OB provider for culture and treatment. This disease, if untreated, may cause blindness in the unborn child.

Hepatitis B and Hepatitis C

Hepatitis B Virus (HBV) can be passed on to the baby if the mother becomes infected during her pregnancy. HBV is transmitted through activities that involve injected drug use, sex with an infected partner or sharing item such as razors or toothbrushes with an infected person. The CDC currently recommends that every pregnant woman undergo testing for hepatitis B. The hepatitis B infection in a pregnant woman poses serious risks to both mother and infant. Without using treatments available for this infection, 40% of infants born to HBV-infected mothers will develop chronic HBV infection and one-fourth will eventually die from chronic liver disease. Identifying hepatitis B infections in pregnant women and providing treatment for the baby within 12 hours of birth can prevent passing this virus to the baby. Discuss this and hepatitis B vaccines (page 18) with your OB provider.

Hepatitis C Virus (HCV) is rarely passed from a pregnant woman to her baby. About 4 of every 100 infants born to mothers with hepatitis C become infected with the virus. The risk becomes greater if the mother has both HIV infection and hepatitis C. To date, there is no preventative vaccine for hepatitis C. The CDC does not recommend routine hepatitis C testing of pregnant women. Pregnant women should be tested for hepatitis C if they currently or in the past injected drugs once or many years ago or received body piercing or tattoos with non-sterile instruments. Hepatitis C testing should be discussed with the OB provider.

Human Immune Deficiency Virus (HIV) and Acquired Immune Deficiency Syndrome (AIDS)

The virus (HIV) is passed from person to person through body fluids such as blood, semen (the male body fluid that contains sperm), and vaginal fluid. Once the virus is in the bloodstream, the virus can invade and destroy cells of the immune system (the body's defense against disease). This damaged immune system leaves the body open for harmful infections that could lead to death. When the body develops this serious infection (AIDS), it lasts for life and almost always is fatal if not treated with antiviral medication.

Pregnant women can give their babies this virus during the pregnancy or at the time of delivery. HIV testing may be offered to you during your pregnancy. Many infected babies die within 3 years after birth. Breast-feeding mothers can also infect their babies through the breast milk. If you think you may have been exposed to the HIV virus, it is important to talk with your OB provider about being tested.

Syphilis

Syphilis is a contagious, long-term, sexually transmitted disease. Symptoms may appear 10 to 90 days after contact. The infected person gets a sore, sometimes painful, on sex organs or mouth. The sore will slowly disappear – even without treatment. Syphilis goes through many stages. About 6 weeks after appearance of the initial sore, symptoms such as low-grade fever, sore throat, sores or rashes may appear. These too, may disappear after a certain time, but the disease has not gone away. In the absence of symptoms, the disease can be diagnosed only by a blood test. Syphilis must be treated; otherwise it will deteriorate the health of the woman, the partner or cause fetal death. If an unborn child is infected; it could be born with heart defects, bone deformities, and other damage that may appear in childhood. Report any suspicious symptoms to your OB provider.

Vaginal Infections

Bacterial Vaginosis

The symptoms of bacterial vaginosis are: vaginal discharge with an unpleasant or "fishy" odor. Redness and itching are rare however, since bacterial vaginosis can occur with other types of infection, other symptoms may be present. In pregnancy, this infection may increase the risk of early labor, delivery or rupture of the membranes (bag of waters). You should see your OB provider to determine what treatment is necessary.

Candidiasis (Yeast)

Candidiasis is caused by a fungus. Although it can affect any woman it is seen more frequently in women who are pregnant, diabetic or obese. Symptoms include: an odorless, white, "cheesy" discharge, itching, burning and redness or irritation of the vaginal tissues. Candidiasis can be treated easily during pregnancy.

Trichomoniasis

Trichomoniasis is caused by a protozoan (one-celled organism larger than bacteria). This type of vaginitis is usually sexually transmitted. A woman may have an irritating discharge, often yellow-green in color. It can also have an offensive odor. The discharge can produce burning and itching, especially during urination, and also redness and swelling. Trichomoniasis is often shared by sexual partners. Successful treatment depends on getting rid of the infection in both partners.

Rest and Exercise

Rest

It is important that you receive adequate rest during pregnancy. Get 8 hours of sleep at night, and take a nap in the afternoon. It is desirable for you to rest on your left side in the later part of pregnancy. This will help control swelling in your feet and ankles and make it easier for your heart to pump blood through your body.

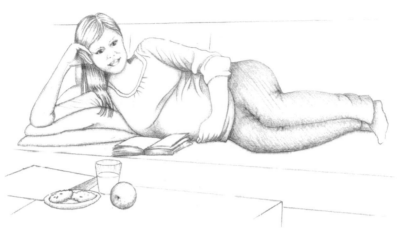

Exercise

You want to be in the best possible shape for your labor and delivery. Although pregnancy is not a good time to begin a new activity, almost any sport that you have been enjoying prior to pregnancy can be continued during this time. If you have any questions regarding your sport, please talk to one of your OB providers. Generally, a "low impact" type of exercise is preferred, such as walking or swimming. If you have not been active in the past, now is a good time to begin a walking program. Start walking slowly and progress to 30 minutes a day. This exercise will help build endurance for upcoming labor and delivery. Walking back and forth at work, chasing after your other children, or shopping is not adequate. You need a program of continuous walking. Try to do this daily, and no less than three times a week. During hot or cold months or rainy days you can drive to a shopping mall and walk around the mall.

Swim if you have access to a pool. Swimming is very good for the legs and abdominal muscles, and for endurance. High impact exercises should be avoided and your pulse should never be above 140 beats per minute.

The exercises on the following pages are helpful in keeping your body in shape while you are pregnant. They will also help relieve some minor discomforts you may experience during pregnancy.

Abdominal Strengtheners

Purpose:
To strengthen and stretch your abdominal muscles and to improve your overall circulation.

Practice:
• Leg Raise - Lie on your back with feet flat on the floor, knees bent. Bring one knee up to your chest as close as you can. Straighten the leg out toward the ceiling. Bend knee and return foot to the floor. Press the small of your back into the floor while doing this exercise. Do the same exercise with other leg. Repeat 10 times each day.

Foot circles can be added to improve circulation.

• Knee Reach - Lie on your back with feet flat on the floor, knees bent. Lift your head and move knee toward nose as close as possible. Alternate legs. Repeat 10 times each day.

• When finished roll to your side to get up.

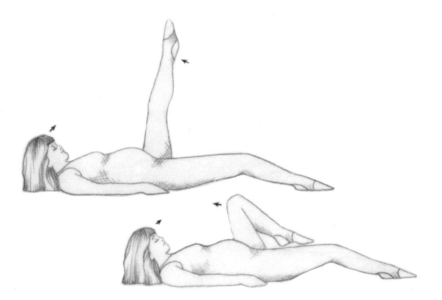

Lying on your back should only be done for the few minutes of exercises. Resting or sleeping on your back places too much pressure against the main blood vessels, possibly interfering with circulation.

Passive Leg Elevating

Purpose:
To promote good circulation in the legs and reduce discomfort from varicose veins, leg cramps, and leg fatigue.

Practice:
• Lie down on left side and elevate legs above the level of the pelvic area using a pillow.

• Do each evening for approximately one hour and when possible, at intervals during the day.

Modified Knee-Chest

Purpose:
To aid in relief of pelvic pressure, hemorrhoids, cramps in the thighs and buttocks and lower back and leg pain.

Practice:
• Kneel, keeping your knees 18 inches apart.

• Place your forearms on the floor. Your pelvis will be higher than the rest of your body.

• Tighten your abdominal muscles slightly in order to relieve the pressure of the baby on your abdominal wall.

• Keep your back straight. Thighs should be perpendicular to the floor. Maintain this position for two minutes, gradually increasing to five minutes.

• Straighten up and relax. Pause before rising to regain your balance.

• Repeat at intervals throughout the day as needed.

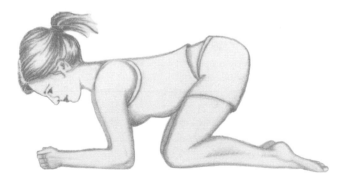

Kegel Exercise (The most important of all!)

Purpose:
To strengthen the muscles around the vagina and to increase the ability to control and relax these muscles completely. This will help prepare your body for labor and a rapid postpartum recovery.

Practice:
• To get the feel of the muscles, stop and start urinating while using the toilet. Practice this tightening and releasing action while sitting, standing, walking, driving and watching TV.

• Try to tighten the muscles a small amount at a time, "like an elevator going up to the tenth floor." Then release very slowly one "floor" at a time.

• Try tightening the muscles from front to back including the anus (rectum) as in the above exercise. Do these exercises every morning, afternoon and evening (three times a day). Start with 5 times each and gradually work up to 20 to 30 each time.

Knee Press

Purpose:
To strengthen your inner thighs, stretch your lower back muscles, and improve your circulation.

Practice:
Sit on the floor; pull your feet (with soles touching) as near to your body as you can comfortably. Keeping your back straight, inhale deeply and press your knees slowly and gently to the floor while you exhale. Hold to a count of 3. Relax and round your back. Repeat this sequence 10 times each day.

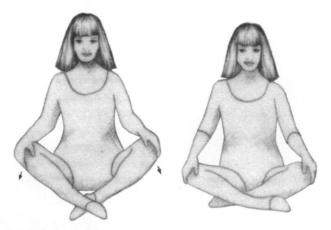

Shoulder Circling

Purpose:
To strengthen upper back muscles and provide relief from upper backache. It also may alleviate numbness in arms and fingers.

Practice:

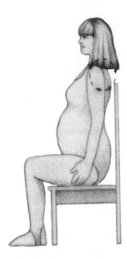

- With arms hanging loosely at sides, lift shoulders up toward your ears.

- Rotate shoulders back as far as they comfortably go.

- Relax shoulders and return to starting position.

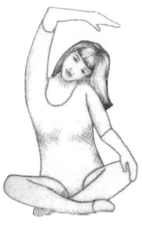

Rib Cage Lift

Purpose:
To relieve pressure under your ribs and make breathing easier.

Practice:

- Curve your arm over your head as high as possible and take a deep breath.

- Alternate and repeat with other arm.

Calf Stretching

Purpose:
To provide temporary relief from leg cramps and, if done regularly, also aids in preventing them.

Practice:

- Stand, placing your hands on the back of a chair with feet together.

- Slide foot of cramped leg as far back as possible without letting the heel leave the floor.

- Bend the knee of the other leg and relax.

- Return to position in step 1 and repeat.

The Pelvic Rock

Purpose:
To strengthen abdominal muscles, relieve backache and improve circulation.

Practice:
This exercise can be done in three different positions. The exercise should be done slowly and done in rhythmical fashion. During this exercise, tighten your abdominal muscles and tuck your buttocks under so that the small of your back is pushed back as far as possible.

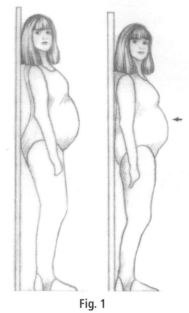

Fig. 1

- Start with your shoulders and buttocks against a wall, knees slightly flexed; "tighten" your buttocks enough to flatten the small of your back against the wall, hold and then relax. If you put your hands on your hipbones, you should feel them rock back and forth with this exercise (Fig. 1). Repeat 10 times.

- Take a position on hands (arms straight) and knees, keeping your weight balanced evenly on them (Fig. 2). Tighten your abdominal (tummy) muscles and tuck hips under. This action will arch your back (Fig. 3). Relax. Repeat 10 times.

Fig. 2   **Fig. 3**

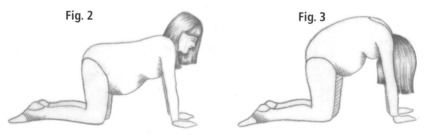

- Lie on your back; bend knees, keeping your feet on the floor. Tighten your lower abdominal (tummy) muscles and the muscles in your buttocks to press the small of your back into the floor. Relax (when you are relaxed, you can slip your hands under the small of your back). (Fig. 4). Repeat 10 times.

Fig. 4

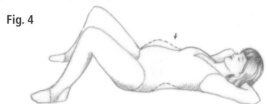

Relief of Common Discomforts

Discomfort	Try this Exercise or Position
Leaking urine when coughing, laughing	Kegel's
Abdominal pain when coughing	Abdominal Strengtheners
Heaviness in pelvis*	Modified Knee-Chest, Kegel's
Hemorrhoids and swelling around vagina	Modified Knee-Chest, resting with hips elevated, Kegel's
Low back pain – one sided*	Modified Knee-Chest
Cramps in thighs, buttocks*	Modified Knee-Chest
Cramps in legs	Leg Elevating, Calf Stretching
Tired legs	Leg Elevating, Calf Stretching
Varicose veins in legs	Leg Elevating, Calf Stretching
Shortness of breath	Good posture, Rib Cage Lifting
Low backache*	Good posture, Pelvic Rock
Middle backache	Knee Press
Upper backache	Good posture, Shoulder Circling
Numbness in arms and fingers	Lying on one side, Shoulder Circling

*See "Pre-Term Labor," page 48

Prenatal Testing

Several laboratory tests are done to obtain information needed to monitor you and your developing baby's health. Listed below are a few of the most common tests used. Your OB provider may omit or add tests to these depending on your pregnancy.

Prenatal Profile: Done on or soon after first OB visit.
• Blood tests:

Blood type and Rh factor (+ or -).

Rubella status to see if you are immune to the German measles.

Hepatitis B virus test to see if you are a carrier of this liver-damaging virus that could be passed on to the baby.

Hepatitis C if you have tattoos or piercings.

Complete blood count (CBC) to see if you are low in iron (anemic). This test is usually repeated several times during the pregnancy.

• Pap Smear to test for cervical cancer.

• Urine screen to test for possible infection and how the kidneys are working.

• Syphilis test (VDRL, RPR) to determine if you have this infection. If so, prompt treatment is necessary. The test may be repeated during the last three months of pregnancy.

• Gonorrhea and Chlamydia culture to detect an infection, necessitating prompt treatment.

• HIV test is recommended in order to detect if you have been infected.

• Other blood tests or cultures may be done depending on your provider.

Genetic Testing:
Your OB provider may suggest the possibility of genetic testing due to your age or a family history of birth defects.
• Non-Invasive Prenatal Testing (NIPT) is a new blood test taken from a mother's arm to screen for some of the most common fetal chromosome abnormalities such as Down's Syndrome (Trisomy 21). This test can be done after 10 weeks of pregnancy and additional texting may be needed if results are positive.
• Chorionic Villi Sampling (CVS): This procedure is done at approximately 9-11 weeks gestation. A small catheter (tube) is placed through the cervix under ultrasound guidance and a small sample of placental tissue is collected. This test also has risk to the pregnancy and should be discussed with your OB provider. This test can detect various fetal problems such as Down Syndrome, Tay-Sachs disease and cystic fibrosis.
• Amniocentesis: This is usually done at approximately 14-19 weeks of pregnancy. A needle is placed, with ultrasound guidance, into the amniotic sac and a small amount of fluid is withdrawn. The fluid's cells are grown and the cells are examined for chromosomal abnormalities. This test does have risks to the pregnancy and must be discussed with your OB provider.

Combination Screening or First Trimester Screen: Done between 10 and 13 weeks. This is the earliest, noninvasive screening test for Down syndrome, Trisomy 18 and Trisomy 13. This is a screening test. If positive additional testing such as amniocentesis may be offered for a more accurate diagnosis. This test involves obtaining blood from the mother and performing an ultrasound on the baby.
- The blood test from the mother measures pregnancy associated plasma protein A (PAPP-A) and free beta human chorionic gonadotropin (hCG)
- The ultrasound test is called a nuchal translucency screening and measures the thickness on the back of the baby's neck.

Triple Screen: Done between the 15th and 20th week.
This test helps your OB provider determine if your baby might have Down syndrome or other problems. It includes the Alpha-Fetoprotein (AFP), a pregnancy hormone called human chorionic gonadotropic (HCG) and estrogen. This is a screening test, further testing may be needed.

Alpha-Fetoprotein (AFP): Done between the 15th and 20th week.
Testing for Alpha Fetoprotein (AFP) is done by drawing a blood sample from your arm. AFP is a protein normally produced by the fetus and present in the mother's blood during pregnancy. In some conditions, AFP levels can be too high or too low, indicating possible spinal or genetic defects. Screening the mother's blood for an elevation or lowering in the AFP levels can identify a problem and may require further testing. This is a screening test. Results may be outside the normal range and not necessarily mean there is a problem. Discuss this with your provider.

Ultrasound (Sonogram) Examination: Done usually between the 18th and 20th week. May be ordered at other times in your pregnancy if complications occur. Ultrasound uses high frequency sound waves that are transmitted onto a television screen. It is a non-invasive, painless method of scanning mother's abdomen to determine baby's growth and development, to detect fetal heart motion, to determine placental placement, and to examine the amount of fluid that surrounds the baby. An Ultrasound is a useful tool to evaluate how your pregnancy is progressing.

Ultrasound as a screening method during the course of pregnancy is useful as a baseline in determination of overdue pregnancies and in diagnosing fetal growth variations, in planning repeat cesarean births, and in determining the cause of some bleeding during the pregnancy.

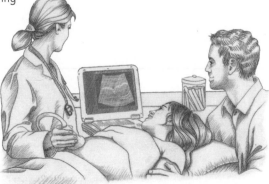

Ultrasound is not used to determine the sex of the baby. To date, there are no known risks and no fetal malformations which have been associated with the ultrasound.

Diabetic Screen: Done between the 24th and 26th week of pregnancy. Pregnancy affects the way some women's bodies use sugar. It may result in a condition called "Gestational Diabetes." If untreated, this can put you and your baby at increased risk. The Diabetic Screen is done to identify these women.

RH Negative:

A woman is either Rh+ or Rh-. If your blood is Rh-, and the father of the baby has Rh+ blood, there is a chance that the baby could have its father's Rh type of +. A small amount of the baby's blood could come in contact with your blood. If this occurs, your body doesn't recognize the + blood type and tries to fight against it by producing antibodies. To determine if this has occurred, a blood test is done between 26-28 weeks to see if you have developed any antibodies against your baby's blood. If this has not occurred, an injection of Rhogam is given to prevent this from happening. You will need Rhogam if you are Rh- and you:

- are between 26-28 weeks in the pregnancy.
- have a miscarriage or abortion.
- are within 72 hours of delivery and the baby is Rh+.
- have an amniocentesis.
- have spotting or vaginal bleeding during the pregnancy.
- have a fall, motor vehicle accident or abdominal trauma.

Fetal Heart Rate Monitoring:

These tests are used to monitor the baby's heart rate and can show how well the baby is getting oxygen through the placenta. Fetal heart rate testing may be done for a number of reasons. Some of these may include: abnormal amniotic fluid level, inadequate growth of the baby, decreased baby movement, elevated blood pressure of the mother, diabetes of the mother or when the pregnancy goes over the due date. There are two types of fetal monitoring, the non-stress test (NST) and the contraction stress test (CST).

- Non-Stress Test (NST): This measures the baby's heart rate in response to its own movements. When the baby moves, its heart rate usually increases. This test usually takes 20-30 minutes, but may take longer if the baby is sleeping. This test may be done once or twice a week.

- Contraction Stress Test (CST): This measures how the baby's heart rate reacts to contractions. These contractions may be produced by having the mother stimulate her breasts or by giving medication into the vein. A normal response to this test suggests that the baby is receiving enough oxygen at the moment.

Biophysical Profile:

This test combines an Ultrasound with fetal heart rate monitoring. It records the baby's breathing, movement, muscle tone and heart rate. It also measures the amount of fluid around the baby. The higher the score the better the baby's condition.

Group B Streptococcus (GBS):

This type of bacteria is naturally found in the mouth, digestive, urinary, or reproductive tract of some men and women. This GBS bacteria "colonization" (a place where GBS is found) usually does not cause any danger to a woman's health, and is not contagious between adults. However, GBS bacteria can be passed from the pregnant mother to the baby during the birth process and can make the baby seriously ill. Pregnant women are usually tested for GBS bacteria between 35-37 weeks of pregnancy. A sample of mucus is taken and sent for evaluation during a pelvic exam. If the results are positive for GBS bacteria, your OB provider may suggest using antibiotics late in your pregnancy or during labor.

The Stages of Pregnancy

Growth of the Baby

1st Month
(0-6 weeks)

This section contains a brief month-by-month description of what is happening to you and your baby as your pregnancy progresses. Be sure to review your responsibilities for each month.

Your Baby

By the end of this period your baby has grown from about ¼ to 1 inch long inside a

sac of amniotic fluid (bag of waters). • Hereditary characteristics were set from the moment the mother's egg (ovum) and the father's sperm met. • Father's sperm has already determined your baby's sex. • Brain and nervous systems are forming. • Heart and lungs are beginning to form. • Tiny spots for ears, eyes and nose are appearing. • Arm and leg buds are forming.

AT THE END OF
FOUR WEEKS

Your Body

You were two weeks pregnant when you missed your first period, and you've already been pregnant six weeks when you missed your second period. • Your breasts now begin to feel tender and tingly. • Your pregnancy test turned positive on the first day of your missed period. • You may feel nausea ("morning sickness") but it can come any time of the day. • You haven't gained weight or changed your body size this month. The placenta is forming and beginning to produce hormones that prepare your body for pregnancy. • You may feel unusually sleepy and tired. • Your uterus will grow larger, softer and rounder, but is down behind the pubic bone where you can't feel it.

Your Responsibility

Make an appointment to begin prenatal care. • Check with your OB provider before taking any medications. • Avoid cigarettes and alcoholic drinks; avoid drinking colas, teas and coffee that have caffeine. • Avoid having any X-rays now that you are pregnant. • Eat a balanced diet of whole-grain breads and cereals, fruits and vegetables, milk products and meat, fish or other sources of protein. • Discuss with your partner any positive or negative feelings you both have about this pregnancy. • Decide how and when you want to tell your family and friends, and maybe your employer, about your pregnancy. • Enroll in early Prepared Childbirth Education Classes.

2nd Month
(6-10 weeks)

Your baby grows to be about 2 ¼ inches long and weighs about ½ to 1 ounce by the end of this month.

Your Baby

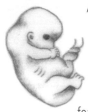

A distinct umbilical cord has formed. • Its head is large because its brain is growing faster than its other organs. • Its heart beats. • Its stomach, liver and kidneys are forming. • This is a critical period in developing your baby's structures for seeing and hearing. • Cartilage, skin and muscles are starting to give shape to your baby's body. • Its fingers and toes are forming. • Its fingernails are beginning to appear. • Its facial features are forming.

AT THE END OF
EIGHT WEEKS

Your Body

The placenta continues to grow and make more hormones. • Your breasts increase in size and the area around your nipples begins to darken. • Your vaginal secretions are becoming thicker, whiter and stickier; the tissues in and around your vagina are bluish from the heavier blood supply brought in to nourish the baby. • Your growing uterus crowds into the space next to your bladder and you begin to urinate more frequently. • You may still have nausea and it may be more noticeable in the morning. • You may still be sleepier and more tired than usual. • Your waistline may begin to get bigger. • Your uterus is still small enough to lie behind your pubic bone but it is softer, rounder and larger now; it may feel like a small lump above your pubic bone by the end of this month. • You may gain a pound or two by the end of this month.

Your Responsibility

Get a prenatal checkup this month and plan to have them regularly. • Ask for your prenatal test results such as your blood pressure, weight and urine each time. Record these in your "Appointment Record" at the front of the book. • Know your blood type and Rh factor. Record this in your "Appointment Record" at the front of the book. • Ask for your hemoglobin or hematocrit results to know if you are low in iron. • Rest and relax; you won't need this much sleep later. • Start a daily habit of exercise - walk, swim, low impact aerobics. • Avoid cigarettes, alcohol, caffeine, junk foods and any medications unless prescribed by your OB provider for use during pregnancy. • Take prenatal vitamins and iron as prescribed. • Eat a balanced diet - plenty of whole-grain breads and cereals. • Try to enroll in an early Prepared Childbirth Education Class. • Share with your partner your ideas and worries about how pregnancy is affecting the both of you because everyone has some feelings of doubt. • Talk with good friends or family members who are parents about their experiences in the first few months of pregnancy. • If you have insurance, find out what maternity and baby benefits you have.

3rd Month
(10-14 weeks)

Your baby measures about 6 inches long and weighs about ¼ pound by the end of this month.

Your Baby

Amniotic fluid around your baby equals about 1 cup. • Your baby swallows amniotic fluid and its tiny kidneys return the fluid back into the amniotic sac. • The umbilical cord is well formed and blood is circulating between your infant and the placenta. • Your baby can move but it is still too tiny to be felt by the mother. • Its heart beats 120 to 160 beats per minute • Your baby's vocal cords are formed. • The sex organs are developed. • By the end of this month, your baby's ears, arms, hands, fingers, legs, feet and toes will be completely formed. • Reflex movements allow your

AT THE END OF TWELVE WEEKS baby's elbows to bend, legs to kick and fingers to form a fist. • Its taste buds are forming. • Its neck is well defined and its head (still the largest part) can be held erect.

Your Body

Your weight gain has been small so far - probably about 2 to 3 pounds. • Your appetite may begin to increase by this time. • Your nausea begins to be more infrequent. • You may notice some tendency to become constipated as hormones of pregnancy cause your bowel activity to be more sluggish. • You may sweat more easily than usual. • Your uterus is now big enough to be felt above the pubic bone; you may even notice it gets hard from a contraction. • The placenta is now completely formed and hormones are produced in amounts needed to keep your pregnancy healthy. • You'll begin to feel more energetic by the end of this month. • Pregnancy may seem like a more stressful time of feeling all sorts of emotions; you may be happy and sad without any good reason.

Your Responsibility

Get your prenatal checkup this month. • Eat a balanced diet with plenty of protein, fresh fruits and vegetables. • Drink at least 6 to 8 glasses of water each day. • Avoid cigarettes, alcohol, caffeine, and any unprescribed medication. • Get some exercise every day - work up to walking 30 minutes each day. • Avoid using paints (except latex), pesticides and aerosol sprays during your pregnancy. • Examine your budget and begin to set aside some money for baby items. • Ask about any changes in your body that worry you. • Allow yourself and your partner to adjust to both negative and positive feelings about this pregnancy; besides your partner, you may want to have someone else you can share all of your feelings with who won't laugh at or judge you. • Decide on feeding method and start reading.

4th Month
(14-19 weeks)

Baby will measure about 10 inches long and weigh about three-quarters of a pound by the end of this month.

Your Baby

The amniotic fluid increases a lot this month and your baby enjoys moving about freely inside the amniotic sac. • Its kidneys now make urine. • Hair begins to appear on its head. • A fine, downy hair (lanugo) begins to appear over your baby's body. • Its eyebrows and eyelashes begin to grow. • Its skin begins to fill out with fat. • It starts a growth spurt in both length and weight. • Baby's movements may become strong enough for some to be felt by the mother by the end of this month.

Your Body

Your uterus grows to just below your navel by the end of this month. • Your weight starts to increase by about ¾ to 1 pound a week now; you may gain about 3-4 pounds this month. • The placenta secretes hormones into your body that help to soften some of your joints and muscles to make labor and delivery easier. • Your appetite increases, so you may be hungry more often. • Cravings may start for certain foods but do not indicate a need for that food. • Your nipples and the area around them become much darker in color. • A line down the middle of your abdomen may darken (linea nigra). • You may have some tendency now to become more susceptible to urinary tract infections, so you need to drink 6 to 8 glasses of water each day. • Your pregnancy is now beginning to show. • You are less tired and fatigued now; you may find you are beginning to enjoy being pregnant.

Your Responsibility

Get your prenatal checkup this month. • Continue to eat a balanced diet with plenty of fruits and vegetables. • Avoid caffeine drinks, cigarettes, alcohol and medications (unless prescribed). • Get some regular exercise; work up to walking at least 30 minutes a day if you have had no pregnancy complications so far. • Make sure that seat belts fit low over your hips. • Learn and practice the Kegel and Pelvic Rock exercises every day. • Lie down with feet slightly elevated on a pillow for at least 30 minutes a day. • Continue to take your prenatal vitamins and iron if prescribed. • Pick out some comfortable clothes to wear as you change size. • If you are employed, find out the procedures for maternity leave. • Talk with your partner about what you both think the baby will be like, its sex, hair color, eye color, personality and also about what it will be like to be responsible for a new baby.

5th Month
(19-24 weeks)

Your baby will weigh about 1½ pounds and be about 12 inches long by the end of this month.

Your Baby

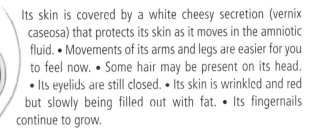

Its skin is covered by a white cheesy secretion (vernix caseosa) that protects its skin as it moves in the amniotic fluid. • Movements of its arms and legs are easier for you to feel now. • Some hair may be present on its head. • Its eyelids are still closed. • Its skin is wrinkled and red but slowly being filled out with fat. • Its fingernails continue to grow.

Your Body

You will continue to gain about ¾ pound a week now or 3 to 4 pounds a month. • Your baby will begin to move a lot; you will notice certain patterns of quiet and activity. • The top of the uterus can be felt at the navel or just above. • Your breasts continue to grow larger; they may get softer and the veins will start to show. • Some women may have colostrum (early milk) leaking from their breasts. • Constipation may become more troublesome now and may continue through the end of pregnancy. • Your hair may begin to feel thicker and oilier. • You usually feel good; people begin to talk about how well you look. • You may have some feelings from time to time of not being able to cope. This can happen almost anytime during pregnancy.

Your Responsibility

Continue your prenatal checkups. • Continue to eat a balanced diet making sure you have enough milk and/or milk products. • Step-up the routine of walking every day and doing the Kegel and Pelvic Rock exercises if you have had no pregnancy complications. • Avoid smoking, alcohol, drugs, junk foods, caffeine drinks and unprescribed medications. Be careful to remember your vitamins and iron supplements (if prescribed). • Drink 6 to 8 glasses of water or other fluids each day. • Take time to purchase one or more well-fitting support bras. • Take time for a rest period on your side every day. (Lying on your back may place too much pressure against the main blood vessels and could possibly interfere with you and your baby's circulation.) • Talk about any concerns you or your partner may have about the responsibilities you will have to assume as parents. • Seek out special friends and family members to help you to deal with your feelings of being nervous as well as sharing the fun and anticipation that goes with having a baby.

6th Month
(24-28 weeks)

Your baby will measure about 14 to 15 inches long and weigh about 2 to 2½ pounds by the end of this month.

Your Baby

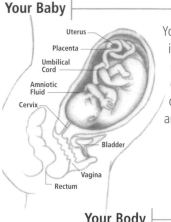

Uterus
Placenta
Umbilical Cord
Amniotic Fluid
Cervix
Bladder
Vagina
Rectum

Your baby can respond to noises from the outside; it may move or become quiet. • It can kick, cry and hiccup. • Its skin is still wrinkled and red. • Its eyelids can now open and close; its eyes are almost completely developed for life outside. • Ridges for fingerprints are forming.

Your Body

You may have occasional heartburn, especially if you eat heavy, greasy or spicy foods. • Your uterus is now felt above the navel. • Your sex drive may increase or decrease; it may change from week to week. • Stretch marks may show up on your abdomen, hips and breasts as you gain weight. • Your weight gain continues to be about 3 to 4 pounds a month. • Your appetite is good; any nausea you may have had should be gone. • You may find yourself dwelling on all the things that can go wrong with your baby. Most women do at some time in the pregnancy. • You find yourself getting more and more involved with your baby as it grows inside you. • You look healthy – there is a special glow to your skin and a sparkle in your eyes.

Your Responsibility

Get your prenatal checkups on schedule even if you feel great! • This is the time you should be thinking about selecting a doctor for your baby. • If you plan to breast feed, schedule breast feeding classes and/or start reading books on breast-feeding. If you plan to bottle-feed, check on what you will need to have in the house. • Take rest periods as needed to avoid drooping at the end of the day; try to lie on your left side and relax (this increases the blood flow to you and your baby). • Continue to eat a good diet with plenty of fruits, vegetables and whole grains. • Start collecting items for the baby's first few weeks. • When family or friends ask, let them know what you and the baby will need. • Talk with other parents about their childbirth experiences; write down questions to ask your OB provider. • Take time to talk about how you feel about your body changes.

7th Month
(28-32 weeks)

Your baby now measures about 16 inches long and will weigh a little over 2½ to 3 pounds by the end of the month.

Your Baby

Its body is now covered with fine, soft hair called "lanugo". • Its fingerprints are set. • It will have definite periods of sleeping and waking. • It moves frequently with noticeable kicking and stretching. • It practices thumb sucking. • Its brain and nervous systems now mature rapidly. • It starts to store iron and will continue until time to be born. • If a boy, its testicles will start to descend into the scrotum.

Your Body

Your uterus is now moving up closer to your rib cage; you may be conscious of kicking against your ribs. • You can watch your abdomen move as your baby moves about. • Your breasts may leak enough to need to wear padding in your bra. • You may notice some swelling of your feet, ankles and hands by the end of the day - especially if it has been hot or you have been on your feet a lot during the day. If the swelling is present in the morning or is extreme, notify your OB provider. • Your weight may tend to increase faster than you expect; this begins the period of the greatest growth for your baby. • You may begin to tire more easily these days. • You may begin to feel a bit more awkward in moving about; you may also notice a bit of light-headedness as you get up from a lying down position. • You may begin to be aware of a loosening in the pelvic bones when you walk.

Your Responsibility

Get your prenatal checkups this month (you probably will have two regular visits this month). • Eat a balanced diet with plenty of protein and iron-rich foods like liver, eggs and meat. • Continue to drink 6 to 8 glasses of fluid a day. • You should not be traveling out of the area anymore. Discuss this with your OB provider. • Practice relaxation and toning exercises each day. • This is the time you should be thinking about selecting a doctor for your baby. • Tour the labor and delivery section of the hospital you plan to use for delivery. • Start thinking about items you will need the first six weeks at home - convenience foods, paper dishes, disposable diapers or diaper service. • Plan some special time with your partner. • Take some extra time for yourself to do things you want to do. • Continue to talk about your feelings, being pregnant and the responsibilities that face both you and your partner. • Begin using fetal movement chart (page 49).

8th Month
(32-36 weeks)

Your baby gains about 2 pounds this month; by the end of the month it will weigh about 5½ pounds and will be about 18 inches long.

Your Baby

All body systems and organs are now mature enough by the end of this month that your baby should be all right if it should be born early, but still needs that extra time of growing in your uterus. • Its skin is smooth as fat begins to fill out the wrinkles. • Its eyes are open. • The soft downy hair gradually disappears. • It is still active with noticeable patterns of sleep and wakefulness. • It may settle down into the position for birth.

Your Body

The top of your uterus is now up near your rib cage. • You may have trouble breathing when the baby pushes up against your lungs. • Your heartburn may increase. • You may have trouble sitting or lying comfortably for long periods of time. • You may have trouble with hemorrhoids. • You can feel the parts of the baby through your abdominal wall. • You begin to tire easily. • You may find this month your most uncomfortable one physically. • Your vaginal secretions increase. • You may sweat more easily. • You may need to urinate frequently day and night as the baby's head crowds your bladder.

Your Responsibility

Plan to get a prenatal checkup every two weeks again this month. • Eat a balanced diet of small, frequent meals. • Drink 6 to 8 glasses of fluid each day. • Continue your exercise program of walking and stretching. • A doctor for your baby should be selected at this time in your pregnancy. • Practice exercises learned in your Prepared Childbirth Education Classes. • Your labor partner and you should be practicing the breathing and relaxation through "pretend contractions" daily now. • Begin to make plans for someone to help you around the house after the birth. • Practice relaxation techniques during Braxton-Hicks contractions (normal tightening and releasing of the muscles of the uterus). • Review what activities will take place during labor and delivery. • Discuss names for the baby with your partner.

9th Month
(36-40 weeks)

Your baby grows 2½ inches and gains 2 pounds - now weighs 6½ to 7½ pounds and is about 20 inches long.

Your Baby

The amniotic fluid equals about 1 quart. • Your baby settles into a head-down position if this hasn't already happened (in most cases). • Baby movements are different since there is less space to move about, but should still be moving as much as it has been. The definite "quiet" and "active" periods continue. (See "Fetal Movement," page 49.) • Its eye color is slate blue, but that will probably change after birth. • Its fingernails become complete and may grow long. • All your baby's body systems and organs continue to mature; it will be ready to take that first breath and grow on its own just as soon as it is born.

Your Body

You see your abdomen getting bigger and wonder how much longer you have before birth. • The Braxton-Hick's contractions are more frequent. • Your abdomen may look lopsided as baby moves arms and legs or shifts positions. • You tire easily and frequently feel drowsy. • Your sleep may be interrupted by the need to urinate and/or change positions. • Your feet and hands may swell. • You may feel pressure low in the pelvis from baby settling into position for birth. • You are tired of being pregnant and ready for delivery.

Your Responsibility

Get a prenatal checkup each week until baby arrives. • Continue to eat a balanced diet. • You may be more comfortable with smaller meals eaten more frequently. • Continue to exercise and practice for childbirth. • Plan now for a birth control method. • Your packing for the hospital should be complete by now. • Set aside clothes for you and baby to wear home if you are not packing them in your hospital suitcase. • List people and phone numbers to call when labor begins. • Take time to treat yourself and your partner to something extra special for the both of you. • Cover your mattress and favorite chair with plastic just in case your bag of waters breaks.

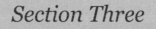

Section Three

Concerns About Pregnancy

Warning Signs

There are certain signs that may indicate possible complications during pregnancy. If any of these occur, report them to your OB provider immediately.

- Vaginal bleeding or spotting.
- Swelling of face, hands and lower extremities (edema).
- Severe continuous headache.
- Dimness or blurring of vision.
- Flashes of light or dots before the eyes.
- Sudden weight gain (more than two pounds in a week).
- Sudden continuous or intermittent abdominal pain.
- Severe or continuing nausea or vomiting.
- Chills and fever over 100.3°F.
- Burning pain on urination.
- Leak or gush of liquid from the vagina.
- Fainting spells or loss of consciousness.
- Decreased fetal movement.
- Suspect labor pains, contractions or rhythmic back pains more than four an hour, if less than 37 weeks pregnant.

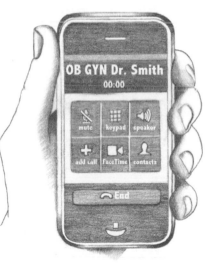

My OB Provider Telephone Number: _____

My Hospital Telephone Number: _____

Pre-Term Labor

Pre-term labor means going into labor before you finish your 37th week of pregnancy.

Pre-term (premature) labor and birth is the largest cause of newborn death and illness today. When babies are born prematurely, they are often small and may have problems with breathing, eating and maintaining body temperature. Some pre-term babies have ongoing illness and handicaps. You need to be aware of the early signs of pre-term labor.

- Dull, low backache.
- Menstrual-like cramps.
- Pelvic pressure.
- Abdominal cramping, with or without diarrhea.
- Increase or change in vaginal discharge.

Contractions:

It is normal for the uterus to contract occasionally. If you feel contractions (tightening of your uterus) more than 4 to 5 times in one hour, you may be in labor. As an example, place your hand on your calf muscle in your leg. As you hold your hand there, first point your toes and feel the looseness of that muscle. Keep your hand on the muscle and slowly pull your toe towards your knee. Feel the tightness of the muscle as you do so. It doesn't hurt to do this. Labor contractions may start the same way; they feel tight but may not hurt.

If you think you may be in labor, don't panic. Lie down on your left side and drink 2-3 glasses of water. If you have 5 or more contractions in an hour, or if the above signs are not gone in an hour, you need to call your OB provider right away. Let them know what you have been feeling and they will advise you. If you are leaking fluid from the vagina and are not sure if it is the membranes (bag of waters), call your OB provider immediately for advice.

If you feel you might be having pre-term labor, be sure to call your OB provider.

If you are diagnosed as having pre-term labor, you will be specifically advised as to the proper care. You may be requested to limit your physical activity, restrict intercourse, get increased rest, modify or stop working, make more frequent visits to your doctor and, perhaps, take medication to suppress labor.

It is important to call or go to the hospital if you have symptoms. If you wait, labor may progress too far and medicine will not stop the contractions or the birth.

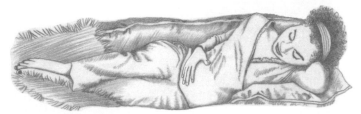

Monitoring Fetal Movement

Recent studies have shown a relationship between fetal (baby's) movements and its health. Daily evaluation of fetal activity will help your provider to identify a potential problem with your baby.

Beginning at 28 weeks (7 months) of the pregnancy, the baby's activity should be monitored by taking the following steps:

• Fetal movement should be counted within 45 minutes after a meal.

• The best time of day to monitor fetal movement is in the evening between 7 and 11 PM. These hours have been selected because babies usually move less during the day.

• Rest comfortably on the left side. You may read, watch television, or do any other quiet activity while you are monitoring your baby's movements.

• Count all fetal movements; these can be any kick, flutter, swish or roll.

• Once you have counted 10 fetal movements, you may go about your usual activity. Record the length of time for the baby to have 10 movements on the sheet below.

• If the baby has not moved 10 times in 2 hours, call your health care center immediately.

Monitoring Fetal Movement			Monitoring Fetal Movement			Monitoring Fetal Movement		
Date	Hour	# Movements	Date	Hour	# Movements	Date	Hour	# Movements

Discomforts of Pregnancy

During the course of a normal pregnancy there are minor discomforts that you may encounter. You cannot always make them disappear, but you can decrease your discomforts if you try some of the hints listed below. If you are not feeling well physically or emotionally with the pregnancy, call your OB provider.

Backache:

Most pregnant women have some degree of backache due to postural changes and ligament stretching and pulling.

Relief Measures: Rest frequently during the day. Maintain good posture. Don't stand in one position or one place too long - shift positions. Use a footstool under your feet while sitting. Wear low-heeled shoes. When picking things up or bending over, bend your knees instead of at your waist. This will cause less strain on your back. The Pelvic Rock (page 28) relieves the low backache. The upper backache is relieved by Shoulder Circling (page 27). If you experience any low, dull backache (that may radiate to side or front) that is rhythmic or constant and not relieved by a change in position, call your OB provider immediately. (See "Pre-Term Labor," page 48.)

Bleeding Gums:

Caused by increased blood volume, swollen mucous membranes and fragile capillaries.

Relief Measures: A dental exam should be a regular part of your prenatal health care. Frequent oral hygiene, increased flossing and "finger massage" of gums will help. If it happens even when not brushing teeth, see your dentist. (See "Dental Work," page 17.)

Breasts:

Begin to enlarge in preparation for lactation and may be tender and even begin leaking. Nipples (areola) may become darker and larger.

Relief Measures: Wear a good support bra. You may find it more comfortable to wear it while sleeping. Your bra should have wide non-elastic straps to provide good support. Wear nursing pads for leaking that are not plastic lined.

Constipation:

This is due to changes in your digestive system. The pressure of the growing uterus may impair the motion of the intestines.

Relief Measures: Eat raw fruits, vegetables, prunes and whole grain or bran cereals. Drink at least 8 glasses of fluid a day. A cup of hot water with lemon three times a day may be helpful. Exercise – walking is especially good. Never hold back the urge to have a bowel movement. Regularity is very important. A "bulk-producing" substance (such as Metamucil, Fibercon or Senekot) or stool softener (such as Colace) may be suggested by your OB provider. Consult your provider before using any medication, or if the symptoms continue.

Difficulty Sleeping:

General discomfort due to any number of "normal" pregnancy symptoms plus inability to get in a comfortable position.

Relief Measures: Do not eat immediately before sleep but drinking milk sometimes helps. Practice relaxation techniques. It may help to go for a walk in the evening followed by a comfortable bath.

Dizziness:

A variety of factors can cause dizziness: Low blood sugar, low blood pressure, standing for extended periods of time and sudden changes of position are a few causes.

Relief Measures: Move slowly when changing positions to avoid creating blood pressure changes, especially if you have been lying down. Eat regular meals. Avoid long exposure to the sun. Discuss these feelings with your OB provider.

Face Pigmentation:

"Mask of Pregnancy" - It is caused by changes in the hormonal levels.

Relief Measures: Experiment with different makeup. Limit exposure to the sun. Usually fades or disappears after pregnancy. A darkened line from the umbilicus down to the pubic area might also be noticed (Linea Negra).

Faint Feeling:

(When Lying on Your Back) - Weight of the pregnant uterus causes pressure on the greater vessels that return blood to your heart.

Relief Measures: Avoid lying flat on your back. If you experience loss of consciousness notify your OB provider promptly.

Fatigue:

Caused by a decrease in the hemoglobin due to a 35 to 50% increase in the blood volume. It is common to feel this early in pregnancy and again the last two months.

Relief Measures: Try to get daily exercise to help prevent fatigue by conditioning your body and improving circulation. Plan to relax by lying down at least once a day. Get plenty of sleep during the night. Do not overdo. Eat well-balanced meals and be sure to take your vitamins. Take iron supplements if prescribed. If your tiredness continues, consult your OB provider.

Frequency of Urination:

The growing uterus presses against the bladder the first months of pregnancy. During mid-trimester the lower segment of the uterus is drawn up, relieving the problem.

Relief Measures: Frequency of urination may be normal. Continue to drink plenty of water. If you have pain with urination or have any low abdominal discomfort call your OB provider.

Headache:

Caused from an increase in circulating blood volume and from the hormone progesterone.

Relief Measures: Try to get adequate sleep, eat a balanced diet and drink plenty of water to prevent headaches. If you do get a headache, try taking a nap, get a massage or try applying warm or cold packs to your temples and forehead. These usually subside after the third month. An acetaminophen product such as Tylenol may be suggested by your OB provider. Call your OB provider if the headaches persist, especially those that appear in the last three months of pregnancy.

Heartburn:

This may occur any time during the pregnancy. It has nothing to do with the heart. It is a burning sensation in the chest or abdomen caused by food backing up from the stomach (reflux).

Relief Measures: Don't lie flat just after eating. However, sometimes lying on your left side or being propped up with pillows may prevent the reflux of food. Avoid heavy, greasy and spicy foods. Try eating smaller amounts of food, but eat more often and drink a small amount of milk or cold water. If it persists, a low-sodium antacid (such as Tums, Maalox or Mylanta) may be recommended by your OB provider. DO NOT take baking soda or any other home remedy. The sodium in these can contribute to fluid retention. Contact your OB provider if your symptoms persist.

Hemorrhoids:

These are varicose veins around the anus and rectum. They are caused by pressure that interferes with circulation.

Relief Measures: Prevention of constipation is important in preventing and treating hemorrhoids. If they protrude through the rectum, you can carefully push them back with a lubricated finger. The Modified Knee-Chest position and hip elevation may help relieve the discomfort (page 25). Practice the Kegel exercise (page 26). Witch Hazel soaks are soothing. Products such as Anusol, Tuck's pads or Preparation H can be purchased at the drug store and may offer some relief from your discomfort. Contact your OB provider if your symptoms continue.

Leg Cramps:

These are generally due to pressure of the enlarged uterus on the circulation of the extremities. They can also be due to the fact that calcium is less easily absorbed during pregnancy. They may occur anytime but especially during the last three months. Leg cramps are not a serious condition but can be very painful.

Relief Measures: Elevate legs frequently during the day. Use a heating pad or hot water bottle for relief. Point toes upward and press down on the kneecap or hold the back of a chair and slide the foot of the cramping leg as far back as you can, keeping the heel flat. This stretches the calf muscle and helps relieve the cramp. Increase calcium (page 12) in your diet. If unable to get adequate calcium from food sources, ask your OB provider about calcium substitutes.

Increased Perspiration:
Activity of the sweat glands is increased.

Relief Measures: Bathing more frequently and changing deodorants sometimes will help.

Nausea (Morning Sickness):
It is not unusual to feel nausea in the beginning of pregnancy.

Relief Measures: Eat dry crackers, toast or cereal before getting out of bed or whenever nausea starts. Eat 5 to 6 small meals each day so your stomach does not get empty. Eating foods in the evening that are high in protein (peanut butter sandwich with a glass of milk) may help. Avoid greasy or spicy foods. Limit your liquid intake during meals but drink water freely between meals. Avoid strong food smells until nausea passes. If nausea persists after trying the above, let your OB provider know.

Nosebleeds:
Caused by increased blood volume, swollen mucous membranes and fragile capillaries.

Relief Measures: May be easily stopped by rest and pressure at the bridge of the nose. If bleeding is frequent and heavy, consult your OB provider.

Pelvic Discomfort:
This can be very common. The growing uterus pulls on the round ligaments, causing pelvic pain. Hormonal influences cause pubic bone and joint relaxation. In the last months of pregnancy, your pelvic joints are movable and this is uncomfortable. Moving fast or coughing may even send a pain up into your abdomen from your pelvis.

Relief Measures: Call your OB provider with any pain or pressure to determine the cause and appropriate care. There are various causes for pelvic discomfort, such as muscle and joint strain, fatigue, excessive weight gain, and pre-term labor. Rest on your left side. Specific exercises such as the Modified Knee-Chest Position (page 25) may help decrease this discomfort. If you experience no relief from the above suggestions, or if you are experiencing rhythmic or constant cramping not relieved by change in position, call your OB provider immediately. (See "Pre-Term Labor," page 48.)

Shortness of Breath:
Difficulty in breathing may be due to the pressure on the diaphragm by the growing baby.

Relief Measures: Moving slowly will help. Lie on your left side, head elevated on more than one pillow. Sometimes sleeping on a lounge chair is necessary. Good posture, rib cage lifting and shoulder circling are of value also. It may be somewhat relieved after "lightening" (baby moves down into the pelvic bones) and will disappear after birth. It is important to discuss this feeling with your OB provider.

Stretch Marks:

They are the result of a breakdown in the lower, less elastic layer of skin. They are also a result of hereditary tendencies. Commonly appear on the lower abdomen, breasts, thighs and buttocks.

Relief Measures: Massaging with lotion will reduce the dryness and itching associated with stretching. Stretch marks fade after the pregnancy but can't be prevented.

Swelling of Lower Extremities (Edema):

Slight swelling of the feet is common and is especially prone to occur in hot weather. It is caused by increased pressure of the uterus on the lower vessels.

Relief Measures: Avoid constricting clothing. Get frequent exercise and drink plenty of fluids. Eat at least three 2-3 ounce servings of protein each day. Lie down when you can and change positions frequently. Try to rest for at least 30-60 minutes daily on your left side with your legs slightly elevated on a pillow. Report any swelling that does not decrease with the above suggestions, or that is present when you wake up in the morning, or any swelling around face or eyes.

Vaginal Discharge:

During pregnancy there are increased vaginal secretions due to the increased blood supply.

Relief Measures: Do not douche. Bathe frequently. Wear cotton panties. Avoid panty hose and/or tight-fitting pants. Avoid vaginal sprays, powders, feminine hygiene products and colored or scented toilet tissue. Vaginal discharge should not be greenish color, foul smelling or irritating. If you have an increase in the amount of mucous or watery discharge, call your OB provider. (See "Pre-Term Labor," page 48.)

Varicose Veins:

These may occur in the lower extremities or extend as high as the pelvis. During pregnancy, the pressure on the abdominal veins by the uterus interferes with the return of blood from the lower legs. If you are constantly on your feet, you will have increased abdominal pressure. The greater the pressure, the higher the tendency of varicose veins.

Relief Measures: You should never wear tight articles of clothing. If possible do not stand in one place for a long period of time (walk about at break time or lie on your left side). Do not sit with your legs crossed or with the pressure of the chair under your knees. Support hose may be helpful and should be put on before getting out of bed. If you have varicose veins around your vagina, try to take frequent rest periods with your hips elevated on a pillow. The Modified Knee-Chest position (page 25) is helpful. If you experience any warmth, redness or tenderness of your groin or legs notify your OB provider immediately.

Intimacy During Pregnancy

Pregnancy should not mean the end of sex! Yet, sex during pregnancy can be an anxiety-ridden experience. It does not have to be. Don't be afraid to have sex during pregnancy. Unless your OB provider determines that there are specific reasons against it, intercourse can be enjoyed throughout pregnancy.

Your sexual relationship has the potential to be more rewarding than ever before. There are new aspects of sexuality for you and your partner to explore during your pregnancy that can make it very special for both of you. Making love, including all the ways you can share pleasure and feel close to your partner, with or without intercourse, is very important to your relationship.

Communication about sex during pregnancy is essential.

The most important thing is not what you feel, nor how silly you think it is, but that you share your feelings with your partner. In this way, you can both make the necessary adjustments for the satisfying sexual relationship.

The following are some answers to questions about sex during pregnancy that commonly trouble expectant couples. Since each pregnancy has its unique qualities, there is no one answer to these questions. Talk with your OB provider about this very important part of pregnancy.

Will sex cause harm to the baby?
Without question the biggest fear during pregnancy - yours and your partner's - is that sexual intercourse will cause harm to your unborn child. Luckily, with few exceptions, sex during pregnancy is considered safe. Nature has provided excellent cushioning for the baby. The fluid it floats in, the membranes (bag of waters) that contain it, the uterus itself, the abdominal wall and the bony pelvis, all help to protect the unborn child from injury.

Warnings about sex during pregnancy:
• Intercourse should be discontinued and seek medical advice if any of the following occurs:
  • vaginal or abdominal pain.   • vaginal bleeding.
  • bag of waters breaks which causes a rush or a trickle of fluid out of the vagina.
  • if you have been diagnosed as having pre-term labor.

• Real caution should be taken concerning anal intercourse. This warning holds as much for before pregnancy as for during. The bacteria from the rectum can quite easily be transferred to the vagina, where they can grow and cause infection. Vaginal intercourse should never follow immediately after the man's penis has made contact with the anal or rectal areas unless a condom is used for one of the acts or a thorough cleansing is done before vaginal entry.

• Man's entire weight should not be placed on the woman, because this can put a great deal of pressure on the uterus and can be quite uncomfortable as the pregnancy advances.

Will my desire or my partner's desire for sex decrease during pregnancy?

You and your partner's reactions to these changes can vary a great deal and may cause an increased or decreased desire for sexual activity. This is perfectly normal.

Both partners have to adjust to these changes and try not to take them personally. Your partner has to make a mental and physical adjustment to a "new" you. You can feel the changes going on inside and outside but he can only guess at them. Discuss these feelings with your partner and encourage him to read about the changes pregnant women experience.

Fatigue, nausea and some other physical discomforts of pregnancy don't always make a woman feel very sexy. Toward the end of pregnancy, a woman can lose interest in sex because all her physical and mental energies are directed towards getting ready for the baby. Your desire for sex may increase simply because you do not have to worry about birth control. Many women experience an increased desire for sex during pregnancy because of the increased blood flow to the pelvis area which causes a woman to become sexually aroused more rapidly and intensely. Many women feel the need for increased affection and assurance that they are loved and still attractive to their partners during pregnancy.

Talk about your feelings with your partner. Sharing honest feelings and concerns is crucial in meeting each other's needs.

Is it harmful to have an orgasm during pregnancy?

Not at all! Orgasm is just as beneficial during pregnancy as it is at any other time. Having an orgasm will make no difference to the baby. Some women late in pregnancy experience continued sexual tension and pelvic discomfort after intercourse because of the increased blood flow to the genitals. Orgasm sometimes fails to relieve this tension. You may find that it takes longer for your body to return to a relaxed state than it did before you were pregnant.

I don't have pain, but the pressure during intercourse causes me some discomfort, what can I do?

If it is simply your partner's weight, this can be taken care of by changing the position. Positions for lovemaking have to be adjusted to your pregnant body. As the fetus grows, you have to try new ways to be comfortable during intercourse. One position that will carry you through most of the pregnancy and avoids the belly-to-belly contact is the side-to-side position with the man behind you so that you fit like a "spoon". Rear entry is good for many couples, especially late in pregnancy, when the woman feels large and uncomfortable. The woman-on-top position is comfortable for many couples especially because she can control the depth of penetration. Late in pregnancy, you may want to choose or explore other positions where penetration is not as deep.

During pregnancy, you and your partner can grow closer together sexually if you realize that not all sex is intercourse, intercourse in one position or having an orgasm. Relax and allow yourself to enjoy these nine special months.

Section Four

Getting Prepared for Delivery

Prepared Childbirth Education Classes

The Prepared Childbirth Classes usually give an overview of the total pregnancy process in order to help the expectant couples gain an understanding of the body changes of pregnancy, the baby's development and the birth process.

Emphasis is placed on breathing techniques and relaxation methods to be used during labor and delivery. Medications used during labor and delivery are usually discussed. What types of medications are used and how much is used will vary widely depending on the person, the labor and the OB provider's medical judgment. The coaches' role is stressed and their responsibilities are very important in labor. The different stages of labor are detailed along with the appropriate breathing techniques for each stage. General hospital policy and procedures may be discussed. A tour of the hospital is an important part of your education for labor and delivery. Also covered should be: when to go to the hospital, how to tell if you are in labor, comfort measures and your responsibilities while in labor and delivery.

There are numerous benefits of taking Prepared Childbirth Classes. Accurate and detailed information is given to help reduce any fears or anxieties you may have about labor and delivery. It is also a time to develop relationships with other pregnant couples as well as enhance your relationship with your partner. Classes are a good time to have questions answered that you may feel uncomfortable in asking your OB provider.

Most classes will use educational videos and written materials to help you understand these complicated events. Many classes are conducted during evening hours to accommodate those who work during the day. Classes usually can be arranged for other work schedules also. Most classes have at least four to six 1-2 hour classes. Being prepared for labor and delivery does make a difference to you and your baby. Register for these classes early in your pregnancy.

Telephone Number for Classes: _____

Date of Classes: _____

Location of Classes: _____

Instructor's Name: _____

Preparing Siblings for the New Baby

Love and trust are two ingredients necessary for healthy relationships. Brothers and sisters of a new baby need to be aware that they are loved and are important members of the family.

Love and trust can be communicated by words and actions.

Some suggestions for preparing brothers and sisters for the new baby are:

• Tell them you love them and the new baby will not change these feelings.

• Take time out to talk and listen to their concerns.

• Involve them in decisions such as names, buying clothes, changing beds, changing rooms, baby-sitting responsibilities, etc.

• Expose young toddlers to new infants by visiting friends, baby-sitting, making a new doll for them to care for or making a picture album of babies cut from magazines.

• Never tell them how lucky they are to be getting a new baby - but how lucky this new baby is to have such a nice big sister or brother.

• Check with your local hospital or community center for "sibling" classes. Change comes over time. The whole family will be changing. Love and trust within the family is the basis for a smooth change.

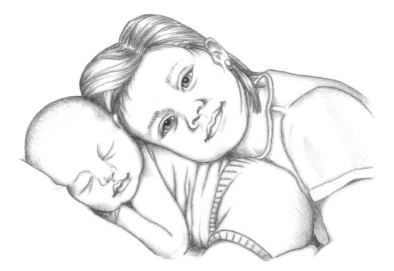

Preparation for the Hospital

Sometime during the eighth or beginning of the ninth month of pregnancy you will want to get together the things you will want to take to the hospital. It is easy to put this off until labor begins but then you will find you do not bring the things you really want or need. Mark on your calendar the day you will pack and then do it. You never really know when your baby will arrive, so be ready at any time.

Here is a list that outlines some of the things you should bring to the hospital. You may want to add your own ideas to this list.

For Mom

Bras - If you are breast-feeding you will find the nursing bra more comfortable. You will need at least two bras. • **Nightgowns** - If you are breast-feeding try to have gowns that open in the front or from the shoulder to make it easier to feed baby. The hospital does have gowns that you can wear. (We suggest you wear the hospital gown at night so as not to stain yours.) • **Bathrobe and slippers.** • **Cosmetics** - Bring the things you need to feel and look good including comb, brush, toothbrush and toothpaste, etc. • **Clothes** for going home - Do not bring tight pants or skirts, as your pelvis will still be a little expanded and your tummy not as flat as you would like. They will not fit. The seam in pants may bother your bottom if you have any stitches. It is best to bring a loose-fitting dress or even wear your gown and robe home. Do not forget undergarments.

For Baby

Diapers, if hospital doesn't supply them. • **Blanket** - With weather in mind decide how heavy a blanket to bring. Remember, even in the hot summer you will need a light cover to shield baby from the sun. • **Nightgown** - Or some other comfortable item of clothing to go home in. Even a shirt is fine, weather permitting. • **Clothes for a picture** - Some like to bring a special outfit for the hospital picture to be taken in. Sometimes this outfit is not very comfortable for baby to go home in. • **Infant car seat** - This is necessary to take baby home.

For Labor Partner

Labor Bag - This can be a cosmetic bag or even a small paper bag. It should contain the things the labor partner needs to help mom in labor. It should have lip moisturizer, lotion (or powder), etc. • **Snacks** - Put things in the labor bag for the labor partner: bottle water, granola bars, hard candy, etc. • List of phone numbers to call after the birth. • **Camera** to record all the events.

Relaxation, Distraction and Breathing During Labor

The following breathing techniques for relaxation and distraction will help you cope with the contractions of labor.

Relaxation

Conscious relaxation keeps your body muscles from becoming tense and tight and helps you stay mentally calm while your body is under the physical stress of labor. It is essential to be comfortable during labor. Practice letting your whole body go limp. (Practice even though that sounds silly.)

• Find the most comfortable position in which to practice. Try using either lying on your side with a pillow between your knees or semi-sitting with a pillow under your knees.

• Work from your feet upward or face downward, relaxing each set of muscles. Become aware of the presence of tension and concentrate on that part of the body until it is relaxed. Include the feet, calves, thighs, buttocks, each vertebrae along the spine, shoulders, upper arms, forearms, hands, neck and face.

• As you become more accomplished in relaxing you should be able to identify tension in your muscles and be able to release that tension to accomplish total body relaxation. Begin by mentally massaging (or your labor partner can massage) each muscle group throughout the body until you are completely relaxed.

Distraction

How do you take your mind off something that is bothering you? Try to find a mental or visual trick that will help you keep your mind off your contractions. Successful distraction can keep a mental focus away from uncomfortable contractions since the brain can only concentrate on one area at a time. Your ability to distract yourself increases your level of overall relaxation.

• Focus eyes on a fixed spot. This might be a picture on the wall, etc.

• Close your eyes and see a calm, relaxing scene: Waves breaking on a deserted beach, clouds drifting across the sky, stream rippling along a meadow.

• Count mentally - numbers, sheep, anything!

Breathing

Get into a comfortable, relaxed position. Breathe in through your nose and out through your mouth with lips relaxed and teeth unclenched. There are many different philosophies that use different techniques of breathing. They all work as long as you work with them. The suggestions below are some techniques we suggest you work with.

• Cleansing Breath - Inhale slowly and deeply. Exhale slowly, slightly forcing the air out. This is a deep, relaxing breath to be done as each contraction begins and ends. It helps you and the baby get a good supply of oxygen. It also helps you relax.

- Slow Deep Breathing - Inhale slowly through your nose and exhale slowly through your mouth. This will be your basic breathing during early labor. Use it as long as possible because it is the least tiring. It lets your lungs expand well and keeps a good supply of oxygen going to you and your baby. It also eliminates muscle tension over the uterus as the uterus tips forward during a contraction. Use a count of "Breathe In-2-3-4, Out-2-3-4..." (This should be approximately a normal resting respiratory rate.)

- Shallow Breathing - In more active labor as your contractions become stronger, last longer and become more frequent, you will naturally begin to breathe faster. These breaths still must be fairly slow breaths to prevent hyperventilation. Therefore by counting "In-1, in-2..." (breathing in on the word and out on the count), you will be breathing at a rate of approximately twice the normal resting respiratory rate.

- Noisy Breathing - Make a "Hiss" or "Whh" sound when you exhale loud enough to hear yourself. Use this in active labor when quiet, rhythmic breathing is no longer enough distraction during a contraction.

- Pant-Blow - Take two quick, short breaths in and then blow out as if you are blowing out a candle. You will use this breathing when you feel the urge to push and it is not yet time. Continue this throughout the contraction and in between if the urge is over whelming. It won't be long until you can push. It is very important not to hold your breath or you will find yourself pushing. Do not push unless you are told to!

- Pushing Breathing - Take two deep cleansing breaths and take a third deep breath and hold it and bear down. Try to push to the count of ten, take a quick breath and resume pushing to another count of ten, letting a thin stream of air flow over your lips as you push to each count of ten. You should be able to get three good pushes with each contraction. You will need to make every push count. It is hard work but very satisfying. While you are pushing, curl your body into the shape of a "C" with your chin on your chest and pulling up and out on your knees. Remember, you only push during a contraction. When it is over, lie back and rest. You need all your strength to push when the next contraction begins.

- Hyperventilation - When you breathe too rapidly the amount of oxygen you take in is decreased and you might get symptoms of dizziness, tingling in the legs, feet, arms or hands and you might feel some confusion. If this happens try to slow down your breathing. During a contraction you can cover your mouth and nose with cupped hands while you continue your breathing. At the end of a contraction you can inhale and hold your breath for a count of 10-20.

Remember
- Distraction helps you relax.
- Relaxation helps you breathe correctly.
- Breathing correctly helps you have the most comfortable labor and delivery possible!

All three of these techniques work together - Not Alone. Though these things seem easy, Practice will help you do them automatically. Practice also gives you confidence!

Labor Summary

The "normal" process of labor and delivery is what numerous women have reported as occurring to them. Many things "expected" to happen in labor and delivery may not. There may also be things that occur to you that are not covered in your classes or in this book. No two women are alike and no two labors that you may have are alike. It is very important to enroll in Prepared Childbirth Education Classes. The following labor information is meant to assist you in your learning and only supplements a formal class situation and your OB provider's medical judgment.

The following changes may occur 2-4 weeks before delivery with a first pregnancy, or in later pregnancies, they may not occur until almost at the time of beginning labor.

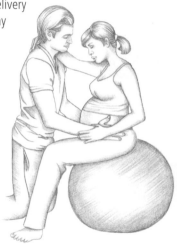

- Settling of the baby deeper into the pelvis.
- Easier breathing.
- Frequency of urination.
- Discomfort from the contractions of the uterus.
- Slight mucus or blood-tinged vaginal discharge (known as "show") may be a week or so prior to labor.

Signs and symptoms of the onset of labor.
- Rupture of membranes (breaking of bag of waters).
- Regular pattern of uterine contractions.

How to time the frequency of contractions:
To time the frequency of contractions, place hand on the uterus and feel when muscles start to tighten. Time from the beginning of one contraction to the beginning of the next contraction.

How to time length of contractions:
To time the length of the contraction, place hand on uterus when uterus is tense (it cannot be indented with fingers). Start timing when the uterus begins to tighten until it begins to soften.

Go to the hospital if you:
- have a sudden gush of fluid or continual leaking of water from the vagina.
- have bright red bleeding.
- are experiencing contractions 5-8 minutes apart, and at least 30 seconds in duration.

Stages of Labor and Delivery

False labor consists of short contractions that do not establish a regular pattern.

Stage One

This period begins with the onset of true labor contractions and ends with complete dilation of the cervix. Total time of the first stage varies from patient to patient. True contractions occur on a regular basis, usually 5 minutes or closer from the start of one contraction to the start of the next. Also the uterus is hard for 30 seconds or more.

Early labor (0-4 cm. dilation)

The baby is descending through the pelvis. The uterine contractions are causing the cervix to efface (thin) and dilate (open).

What you may feel - Uterine contractions (felt as backache, pelvic pressure, gas, menstrual-like cramps, etc.) which may follow a regular pattern and may be accompanied by: (1) rupture of membranes; (2) show (heavy mucus discharge); (3) a sense of relief and/or anticipation.

What you can do - Carry on with normal activities, if possible. Pelvic Rock exercise if back aches (page 28). Time contractions (from beginning of one contraction until the beginning of the next). Use "Slow Deep Breathing" (page 63) if contractions are strong and you are unable to walk, talk or sleep through them.

What others may do for you - Your coach may help time your contractions, offer support and encourage you to relax. Your coach or others may call and get instructions when needed and take you to the hospital if directed. At the hospital, your OB provider takes your pulse, respirations, temperature, blood pressure, baby's heart tones, times contractions, performs a vaginal exam and possibly starts an intravenous in your hand or arm. You may also have a fetal monitor applied to your abdomen to hear the baby's heart beat and measure your contractions.

Active Labor (4-8 cm. dilation)

What you may feel - Uterine contractions will become stronger, last longer and be closer together. They may be felt in: (1) abdomen; (2) above pubic bone; (3) in the back; (4) upper thighs. You may also feel a growing seriousness, a desire for companionship, ill-defined doubts and fears. A "threatened" feeling that things are getting ahead of you.

What you can do - Assume the most comfortable position; try to relax more and more after each contraction. Use your "Slow Deep Breathing" (page 63) with contractions and breathe normally between contractions. Empty your bladder. Try gentle circular rubbing on abdomen with both hands during contractions (effleurage). Ask for medication if needed. RELAXATION IS ESSENTIAL!!

What others may do for you - OB provider continues check of baby's heart tones and mother's vital signs, and pelvic examinations. OB provider should continue to keep you informed of your progress. Coach can help you become more comfortable with: (1) cold washcloth to face and neck; (2) crushed ice if allowed; (3) back rub for back pressure; (4) give you words of encouragement; (5) breathe with you. Ask for other things that make you more comfortable.

Transition (8-10 cm. dilation)

What you may feel - Uterine contractions are at their strongest and about 1-3 minutes apart lasting 50-60 seconds. There may be: (1) amnesia (can't remember things) between contractions; (2) cramps in legs; (3) generalized discomfort; (4) marked restlessness; (5) perspiration on upper lip and forehead; (6) nausea and vomiting may occur, burping and hiccupping; (7) profuse, dark, heavy "show"; (8) pulling or stretching sensation in pelvis; (9) rupture of membranes if still intact; (10) shaking of legs; (11) pressure of the baby's head against the rectal wall and feeling as if you need to move your bowels or that you have to push. DO NOT PUSH UNTIL GIVEN PERMISSION; (12) bewildered by intensity of contractions. Irritable and unwilling to be touched. Frustrated and unable to cope with contractions. Total involvement and detachment.

What you can do - Use in the following order, moving from one to the next only if they are no longer helpful: (1) "Slow Deep Breathing"; (2) "Shallow Breathing" (this is usually automatically done); (3) "Noisy Breathing"; (4) if you feel the desire to push, but are told not to, use the "Pant-Blow Breathing"(page 63). DO NOT HOLD YOUR BREATH. Sleep between contractions. Assume most comfortable position. Realize that pushing reflex is getting ready. Keep in mind that contractions have now reached maximum strength and relief will soon come with pushing. RELAXATION IS ESSENTIAL!!

What others may do for you - Coach can apply cool washcloth to face. Change pads underneath frequently. Back rub or backpressure may help. Much patience and a lot of encouragement. (Remember coach, if you feel you need help, call for your labor nurse.)

Stage Two

This period begins with the complete dilation of the cervix and ends with the birth of the baby. The baby is passing down through the soft tissue of the birth canal, over the perineum and finally birth occurs.

Pushing

What you may feel - Relief because second stage has begun. Pressure to rectum causing a burning or stretching sensation. Total involvement. Exhaustion after each expulsive contraction. Backache, cramping and other discomforts usually disappear as pushing begins. Desire to participate fully or, conversely, to be "put to sleep".

What you can do - Take two "Cleansing Breaths," take another deep breath and hold. Curl your body into a "C" by putting your chin on your chest, rounding your shoulders and pulling your knees into your body and spreading them apart (page 63). Push to the count of 10 then take a quick breath and push again to 10 and, one last time take a quick breathe and push. Long steady pushes bring the baby easier and quicker down the birth canal. Continue pushing throughout contractions. Rest completely between contractions.

What others may do for you - OB provider continues monitoring baby and gives specific instructions with each contraction. Others may hold your head and shoulders up, and urge you to push.

Delivery or Birth Phase

What you may feel - Stretching or burning at vaginal outlet. As baby emerges you may have a burning sensation. The vaginal outlet or bottom (perineum) may tear. Relief follows as the baby is released from your body.

What you can do - Pant or bear down as directed. Listen for the first cry of YOUR BABY!

What others may do for you - OB provider prepares you for delivery: Perineal area is washed; legs, thighs and abdomen are draped with sterile sheets; occasionally an episiotomy is performed to help deliver the baby quickly. Coach can give constant encouragement and directions with each contraction.

Stage Three

This period begins with the birth of the baby and ends with the delivery of the placenta, membranes and umbilical cord.

Pushing

What you may feel - Slight contractions. Exhausted, but elated and proud of achievement. Hungry and thirsty.

What you can do - Follow instructions; you may need to give a little push.

What others may do for you - You will be prepared for the recovery period. If you have had an episiotomy or tear, it will be repaired.

What others may do for your baby - Your baby will have its mouth suctioned out, cord cut and kept warm. An Apgar score will be done on the baby at 1 minute and 5 minutes after birth. A score of 7 or more (maximum of 10) at 5 minutes means baby is in good condition. This score is an indication of how well the baby did during labor and delivery.

Apgar Scale

Item Tested	0	1 Point	2 Points
Heart Rate	absent	slow - less than 100 beats per minute	100 beats or more per minute
Breathing	absent	slow or irregular	regular
Muscle Tone	limp	some motion of extremities	active motion
Skin Color	blue	pink body, blue extremities	pink all over
Reflex Response	absent	grimace	cry

Coach's Reminder Sheet

The coach should be prepared to offer the following support during the various stages of labor.

Early Labor

• Be calm and confident in yourself. Your presence and support are very important contributions.

• If contractions begin at night, and are mild, urge her to get more sleep. If they begin during the day, and are mild, pass the time by reading to her, talking, playing cards, watching TV, etc.

• Do not force her to lie down. Sitting in a comfortable chair with legs supported, alternating with walking, is usually more comfortable. Offer support and encourage her to relax with contractions.

• No special "labor" breathing should be started until she feels the need. Then she should breathe deep, slow and even. At this point she can usually control her breathing with a few words of praise from you.

• Be sure you know the route to the hospital and the approximate time it will take. Be sure your tank has enough gas at all times. Drive carefully and avoid sudden stops and rapid turns. Remind your partner to breathe slowly and evenly with contractions. If you need more than 1 pillow, bring them with you.

Active Labor

• Contractions will be closer, stronger and last longer. She will not want to chat now but will become more quiet and preoccupied with her labor. Do not try to distract her but encourage her as she concentrates on working with her contractions. She will be monitored and may have an I.V. (intravenous) started once she's admitted to the hospital.

• A quiet, subdued environment will aid her ability to relax. Avoid lights shining in her eyes, excessive movement and noise in the room.

• Position is important to her physical comfort and ability to relax. Positions should be changed frequently. There are a variety of positions that can be used such as lying on her side, sitting, walking, squatting, etc. She will usually be more comfortable on her side. One position she should never use is flat on her back. Her legs are usually more comfortable slightly flexed and perhaps with a pillow between them. Be sure the abdomen is also supported if she is on her side.

• Women in labor appreciate little gestures of comfort. A cool wet washcloth to mop her face and neck; cracked ice or a wet washcloth to chew on. A moistened mouth will feel good. Firm pressure to her back eases lower back discomfort.

• Offer frequent words of encouragement. Words like, "You're doing fine," "Wonderful," and "Keep it up" are helpful.

• Help her with her breathing. Her best tool in aiding her to relax and to take attention from the contraction is her breathing. She should be breathing slowly and rhythmically - in through the nose or mouth, but out through the mouth. If you remind her to keep her tongue behind her front teeth, her mouth will not get so dry. (If she has numbness or tingling of the hands, arms, feet or legs, she may be breathing too fast and hyperventilating. Breathing in a paper sack or cupped hands for a few breaths will help.)

- Transition is the most demanding period of labor. Contractions are long, strong and seem to be one right after the other. She may become irritable, discouraged and may momentarily panic. She now needs help more than any other time. She will need some one to give directions with each contraction. (She should go to the bathroom prior to beginning of this stage if possible.)
  - Remind her this period will be short and she will feel better when she can push and should use the rest period between contractions.
  - If she does panic, speak to her in a firm voice saying, "Breathe with me, keep it up, that's good", etc.
  - A catch in her breathing with the urge to push (as if to move her bowels) signals the onset of the second stage of labor (Delivery Stage). Be sure to notify the nurse if she is not right there.

- Second stage will bring mixed feelings of surprise and joy. She needs guidance as to what to do. Be sure you have medical permission to push.
  - When a contraction begins, encourage your partner to take 2 or 3 deep breaths then hold her breath with her lips shut and bear down firmly and steady, letting a thin stream of air flow over her lips. When needed, let out, take another breath and continue pushing throughout the contraction.
  - Hold her head up slightly, have her grasp her ankles or thighs and hold her feet off of the bed when she is pushing.
  - Offer her ice chips and wipe her face with a cool cloth between contractions.

- If you plan to be present for the delivery, you will be asked to change into hospital surgical clothes.

After Delivery

- After she delivers, she will have a recovery period where she will be closely watched. The baby will be weighed. If the father is not present for the delivery, he will be called from the waiting area when mom is in her recovery period.

- After a short visit, you both need a rest. Let her sleep, and you go home and rest. Come back refreshed.

- Ask one of the nurses if a gown must be worn and hands washed when the newborn baby is in the room. Grandparents and the baby's brothers and sisters may also be able to visit mother and baby.

Cesarean Birth

Every pregnant woman should know about cesarean births. It can happen to anyone and the number of cesarean births is rising. About one out of every three or four births is a cesarean. Most mothers having their first cesarean birth have them because of a problem that comes up in labor and are told by their OB provider that a cesarean delivery is needed. Understanding what procedures will take place and the reason for each can make it less frightening. Asking questions during your prenatal visits can help you be prepared if this happens to you.

What is a Cesarean Birth?

A cesarean delivery is the birth of a baby through an incision (cut) in the abdomen and the uterus (womb), after an anesthetic (being put to sleep or given an epidural to keep from feeling pain) has been given to the mother. Antibiotics and modern sterile techniques have made a cesarean delivery one of the safest operations. A cesarean birth protects the health of the baby and the mother in situations that might otherwise be dangerous.

A cesarean birth can be a couple-centered experience - if you are prepared for it. It is not a sign of failure if you cannot have a vaginal delivery. You can still use much of the information you learned in Prepared Childbirth Education Classes. Finding out ahead of time how both of you can be involved in the cesarean delivery can help you be ready.

Why a Cesarean Birth May Be Needed?

• The baby is too big to pass through the mother's bony pelvis.

• The baby's heartbeat shows it is not getting enough oxygen or indicates it is experiencing other signs of distress.

• The baby is in an abnormal position - breech (buttocks coming first), transverse (sideways), etc.

• The placenta is blocking the opening of the cervix (placenta previa).

• The placenta separates from the uterus before the baby is born (abruptio placenta).

• Labor is not progressing adequately.

• The mother has herpes virus of the vagina near the time of delivery.

• The mother is having twins or triplets, etc.

What happens during a Cesarean Birth?

Procedures for a cesarean birth may vary somewhat but the following are considered routine practices:

• A nurse will wash and shave the area where the incision will be made.

• Blood tests will be done to determine your blood type and Rh so blood can be ready if you have unexpected heavy bleeding.

• A catheter (tube) will be inserted into your bladder to drain your urine into a plastic collecting bag. This keeps your bladder out of the doctor's way when the incision is made. This is not a painful procedure. The catheter will be removed the next day.

• An intravenous (IV) needle will be inserted into your arm to allow nourishing fluids and medications to be given. This will assure that necessary nourishing fluids are provided for your body and is generally continued for up to about 24 hours or until you can begin to eat and drink comfortably.

• You may be given an antacid to drink to neutralize acids in your stomach in case you vomit.

• Your abdomen will be scrubbed with warm and then cold solutions and then painted with iodine to get rid of all bacteria (germs) where the incision will be made.

• Either an epidural anesthetic (mother awake but feels no pain) or general anesthetic (mother asleep and feels no pain) will be given, depending on what you, your anesthesiologist and your OB provider decide ahead of time.

• A cesarean takes from 45 to 90 minutes to complete. The baby is delivered within 5 to 10 minutes. Then the doctor lifts the placenta out.

• Then your uterine and abdominal walls are sutured (stitched), which takes most of the time.

• You are given an oxytocic drug to prevent you from bleeding.

There are various types of both skin and uterine incisions. They are not always in the same direction and the decision is up to your OB provider. The abdominal incision may be horizontal (bikini cut) or vertical (up and down or classical). The incision in the uterus may also be horizontal, sometimes allowing a future vaginal delivery, or vertical in which a future pregnancy may have to be delivered by repeat cesarean.

Topics to Discuss During Prenatal Visits

You should talk to your OB provider ahead of time about what options are available if you have to have a cesarean delivery. Topics to consider ahead of time can include: the cesarean birth procedure your OB provider and your hospital use, the presence of the coach in the operating and/or recovery room and breast-feeding on the delivery (operating) table or in the recovery room.

Cesarean mothers can be successful nursing mothers. The sooner a baby begins to suck the better the chances of successful breast-feeding.

"Once a cesarean - always a cesarean" is not always true. Frequently it is safe to deliver your next baby vaginally; however, this must be discussed fully with your OB provider and medical records of your previous cesarean are necessary.

After Cesarean Birth

If the baby is breathing properly (cesarean babies sometimes need extra time and stimulation to begin breathing on their own), and you are awake, you may want to ask if you can hold your baby for a little while and breast-feed. If the coach is in the delivery (operating) room, he/she should be allowed to hold and cuddle the baby too. This is an important opportunity for parents and baby to get acquainted.

Your baby may then be taken to a Special Care Nursery for an observation period. In many hospitals this is standard procedure for all cesarean babies.

You will be transferred to the recovery room following the delivery and will remain there until the anesthetic wears off. This may take from 2-5 hours. Some hospitals allow coaches and/or babies to stay with you in the recovery room. After recovery you will be moved to a postpartum area where other new mothers are. Pain medications will most likely be available following the surgery.

The sutures or small skin clamps are usually removed about the 2nd day (some doctors use sutures [stitches] that dissolve). Your physical condition at the time of surgery and the reason for the cesarean section will be the major factor in how quickly you recover and when you will be discharged from the hospital.

Remember a cesarean is simply one of two ways to have a baby.

Recovery After Cesarean Birth

There are exercises that can be done while you are still in bed that will help prevent complications, reduce gas pains and speed up recovery. They take some effort but are worth it. Ask your OB provider about these exercises.

Rest is vital for your recovery. For 2 to 3 weeks after you go home you should have live-in help; a relative, friend or your partner to take over household tasks. Until the baby is a few days old, you should try never to be left alone. You will probably be in bed much of the time for most of the first week except to go to the bathroom and to care for your baby. From the end of the first week to the third week, you should be up daily with frequent rest periods but avoid taking over regular household tasks of lifting anything heavier than your baby. Remember that over-doing when you begin to feel better will only delay your getting back to normal.

The scar from the incision will fade but will not disappear completely. If a cesarean birth is done with the next baby the same incision site is usually used and the old scar tissue removed.

Don't be afraid to hold, touch and enjoy your baby as soon and as much as possible. This helps the mother and baby start enjoying a new, healthy life together.

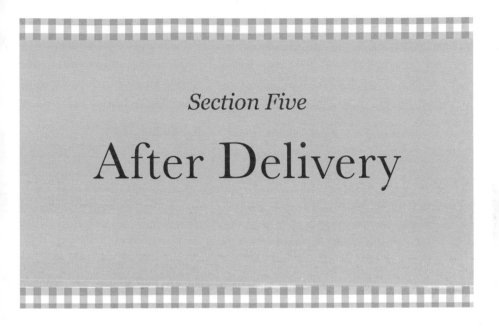

Section Five

After Delivery

Breast or Bottle-Feeding

One of the many decisions you must make regarding the care of your newborn is how you will feed your baby. Before you decide, here are some facts to consider:

Breast-Feeding

Breast milk is ideally suited for the newborn:
- It meets babies nutritional needs from birth through the first year of life.
- Your antibodies help protect baby against some diseases. This is temporary, so babies will need their own immunizations later.
- Factors in breast milk help clear the intestines of meconium - the first dark bowel movements the baby will have. It helps protect against diarrhea and intestinal disorders.
- It provides an extra closeness between you and your baby.
- It digests easier than formula.

It promotes recovery for you:
- The hormone released while feeding contracts the uterus and returns it to normal size quicker.
- Prolactin, the "mothering hormone," may foster closeness to your baby.
- It burns calories. The extra weight gained will be lost faster if you breast-feed.

Convenience and cost:
- Breast milk is always available, clean and warm, and ready for baby. No bottles to prepare.
- Less costly than formula.
- Breast milk can be pumped and put into bottles.
- Progestin-only pills (mini-pills) or contraceptive injections (Depo-Provera) may be used for contraception while breast-feeding. Discuss with your OB provider.
- Returning to work does not prevent you from breast-feeding.

Bottle-Feeding

There are some reasons a woman may prefer bottle-feeding.
- Bottle-feeding allows others to feed baby.
- There is no problem taking certain medications, such as a birth control pill.
- Formula is available at most local stores.
- Formula is available in ready-to-feed cans or bottles. However, powder provides the same nutrition at less cost.
- Cow's milk should be avoided during the first year.
- It may seem more convenient.

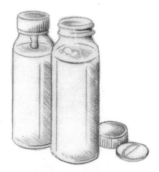

One Day After Delivery

Talk with your partner and friends about your labor and delivery experience.

Your Baby

Your newborn baby may look wrinkled and red. • Its head will be large compared to the rest of its body. • Its head may be a bit out of shape from moving through your birth canal. • The top of its head will have fontanelles (soft spots) in front and in back. • Its eye color will be slate blue, but will probably change. • Its breasts (both sexes) will be swollen from your hormones, but this goes away in a few days. • A boy baby may have a swollen scrotum. • A girl baby may have a slight bloody vaginal discharge. • Your baby can focus on your face, respond to your voice and your touch. • It can grasp your finger, suck its own fingers, nurse and capture everyone's attention with its own special, endearing, newborn qualities.

Your Body

You will have a vaginal discharge (lochia) of blood, mucus and tissue from the uterus that may last 1 to 5 weeks after birth. • If you have an episiotomy incision (a cut made to make it easier to deliver the baby) or a tear, this area will be sore and tender. • You may have some difficulty urinating at first because of tissues being swollen. • Milk will not come into your breasts right away, but the colostrum will provide enough nourishment for your baby. • You may sweat profusely; this is a way nature helps you get rid of excess fluids stored naturally during pregnancy. • You may feel both fatigued and elated. • Your abdomen continues to be large and flabby until your muscles have time to tighten up again. • You will lose weight gradually as the stored fluid is lost through frequent urination. • You will want to eat, sleep and bathe. • You want to be close to and cuddle your new baby. • You want to share all the joy and excitement of birth with your mate.

Your Responsibility

Repeat Kegel exercises (page 26) right after birth and continue them 3 to 4 times daily. • Get up and walk as soon as you are told you can. • Drink lots of liquids and eat when hungry. • Rest whenever you feel tired. • To increase the milk flow, breast-feed your baby as soon as possible after delivery and at least every 2 to 3 hours (whenever baby is hungry). • Hold your baby so his/her bare skin touches yours - hold, cuddle, touch and enjoy your baby.

Postpartum Period
After the Birth

After nine months of getting used to the pregnant you, you are a nonpregnant woman again - a MOTHER!! Regardless of how much you want the baby, how ready you are for it, and how positive your birth experience may be, it is still a big change and adjustment for you to make in your life.

All of the changes in your body that occurred gradually over a nine-month period must now begin to change back. No matter how good you may feel, you should still be kind to your body and take it easy. In addition to undergoing these major physical changes following the birth of your baby, you will also have emotional reactions to the new state of motherhood. These may be either positive or negative and most likely a little bit of both. A "feeling of motherhood" is something you may not have right away. It takes time for you and your baby to get to know each other.

If you really work at it, you will find that there is an almost limitless list of things you can worry about in the postpartum period. So right from the start, try to keep yours to a minimum. Here are a few suggestions to help you prepare and adjust to this period just after birth.

Find Someone to Talk with to Share Your Concerns
This may be someone in your Prepared Childbirth Education Class. You can arrange to get together with some of the women from your classes after you all have given birth. You are all going through the same stage of adjustment together and just knowing you aren't alone is a big help. Often your best source for tips is other mothers who have had experiences with babies.

If you feel you may harm, abuse or neglect your baby - seek help!

Try to be Realistic About What to Expect in a Newborn and What the Initial Postpartum Period Will Bring
Be prepared to be unprepared! Even if you have heard how rough it is going to be the first few weeks, you will most likely underestimate the responsibilities. Some first-time parents have never seen a newborn baby. Each baby is unique and there are normal variations. Most newborns do not look like they do in the advertisements. You may not understand why your baby cries or doesn't smile back at you. Ask your friends who are parents what their baby looked like and how the baby acted the first few weeks after birth. If you are concerned about anything, discuss it with your pediatric provider. When you first bring the baby home, you may feel that you are not exactly sure how to take care of a newborn. Be patient - you will learn by experience. All parents have to be "first timers" at infant care. Don't be afraid to admit your concerns about parenthood.

Do Not Ignore the Signs of Fatigue
Many women are surprised by just how tired they feel both emotionally and physically in the first few months or so. Tune into the signs that your body gives you about being tired or having little energy. Relax and enjoy this period with your baby.

Sleep is essential in the postpartum period. Go to bed early. Try taking a nap or resting when the baby naps. Have a sign on the door stating "Mom and baby asleep" so unexpected visitors will not wake you. Unplug the phone during a rest period.

Try to Limit Your Visitors the First Few Weeks
Everyone will want to see the new baby and this can tire you out very fast. Spacing the time between visitors will help. If you want company, do not try to be a super hostess. (They can get a drink for themselves from the kitchen and there is no reason for them not to get one for you while they're up!) Often friends want to help out but they don't really know what to do to be of assistance - so tell them.

If People Offer Help - Accept It!
Although it may be possible for you to manage by yourself, it will be a great deal easier to have an extra pair of hands. You may want a family member, a close friend or other reliable person to help you with some of the household chores. This is a good opportunity for the father to show off his housekeeping skills and to practice taking care of the baby. For the first week or two, the father can cook, clean, answer the phone, fend off visitors and run errands. You don't actually need help to care for the baby (whose needs are basically to be fed and changed) because this is a special time for you and the baby to be together. Accept the fact that certain things will go undone for a while.

Avoid lifting any heavy objects (heavier than the new baby) and climbing stairs any more than is absolutely necessary the first few weeks.

You May Become Depressed for No Obvious Reason
It is perfectly normal to feel tired, blue and a little let down after the excitement of pregnancy and delivery. It usually lasts no longer than a day or a few weeks and is marked by tearfulness, anxiety, depression, restlessness and irritability. There are times you may be frustrated, resentful or angry. Your hormones are in a state of flux after the birth of your baby and are a major reason for this emotional unpleasantness. The lack of uninterrupted sleep, your changing role with your mate and the baby's constant needs all contribute to the "Postpartum blues." "Postpartum blues" is no joke. If you find yourself depressed or unable to cope with your changed life after the baby is born, discuss your concerns with your OB provider and get some outside help right away. If you don't do this, your depressed state can become even deeper and can have dangerous effects on your physical health and may affect your relationship with the baby and your mate.

Weight Loss After Birth is Something Most Women Welcome
It is normal to lose up to 20 pounds the first week after birth. Although you will have more weight to lose, do not go on a strict diet right away - diet later! Even if you are not breast-feeding, your body requires a nutritious well-balanced diet in order for you to maintain good health and to keep your energy up.

About seven pounds of fat were stored to give you an energy reserve for about the first three months after birth. Assuming you eat properly and get adequate exercise, these extra pounds will gradually drop off.

If you are breast-feeding, nutrition is very important to you and your baby. The nutrients your baby receives while breast-feeding depends on the quality of your diet.

Two is Company, Three's a Crowd?

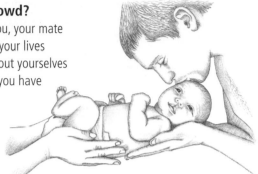

Think of the cliché as it applies to you, your mate and the baby. Having a new baby in your lives changes the way both of you feel about yourselves and how you relate to each other. If you have other children, it is often hard for them to accept a new baby that will be taking the major portion of their mother's attention in at least the first few weeks.

Adjustment to each of your roles is important. Many couples feel anxious about coping and are overwhelmed by the responsibilities of caring for a newborn. Couples who discuss and agree on ways to share and divide basic family responsibilities have an easier time adjusting. Your ability to communicate with each other can prevent some problems and solve others.

Postpartum Priorities

After the birth of your baby, there will be many demands on your time and attention. Advice will come from everywhere – friends, relatives, magazines, TV, etc. You may have a vision of a perfect home with a content baby, happy husband, sparkling floors and baking bread. These things are all possible but keep your expectations reasonable. Remember, "supermom" only exists in the movies. Find out what is important to you and your partner - ESTABLISH YOUR PRIORITIES!

Take some time for yourself each day to read a magazine, polish your nails, exercise or whatever interests you. A few minutes each day spent on your own interests can make the difference between contentment and depression.

Meals are a necessity but often occur when the baby is fussy. During the last months of your pregnancy, double your recipes and freeze half of each. Collect recipes for casseroles that usually contain meat, vegetables and rice or pasta. This is a meal in itself, and can be made during the day and then refrigerated until you put it in the oven. Remember, there is nothing wrong with disposable plates, utensils and oven dishes. They are timesaving!

Juggling baby care, personal relationships and household chores can be a difficult feat. The mark of a seasoned mom is to plan ahead, learn some tricks of the trade, use your time wisely, and then, ROLL WITH THE PUNCHES!! There will be good days and there will be bad days, but remember, both your baby and your partner want you to be a happy and smiling person. Enjoy these precious years and before you know it, you may find yourself giving baby care advice to all your expectant friends.

If You Are Not Feeling Well, or Experiencing Pain Anywhere, Notify Your OB Provider

Do not wait for the post-delivery checkup if you are not feeling well or experience pain anywhere. Although it is common to feel tired, you should not feel ill after birth. If you have any of the following problems; call your OB provider at once.

• Unusually heavy or sudden increase in vaginal bleeding (more than a menstrual period or if you soak more than 2 sanitary napkins in an hour).

• Severe depression or feeling you may hurt yourself or your baby.

• Vaginal discharge with a strongly unpleasant odor.

• Specific area of extreme tenderness in the stitch area.

• Pain, redness, tenderness and/or swelling of your legs (edema).

• Loss of appetite for an extended period of time.

• A temperature of 100.3°F or higher.

• Breasts are red and/or feel painful.

• Pain in your lower abdomen or back.

• Constipation.

• Pain or burning on urination.

• Inability to urinate.

• Persistent headaches.

• Dizzy spells.

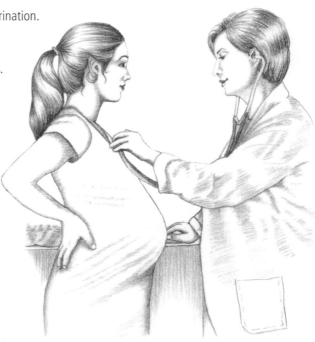

Intimacy
After Delivery

How soon after delivery can sexual intercourse be continued again?

Your body has many changes to undergo after birth, all of which can affect your sex life. Your hormones must readjust to pre-pregnancy levels. Your uterus and vagina have to return to their normal size. It is usually recommended that you wait until after your post-delivery checkup 6 weeks after delivery and you are told all is healed.

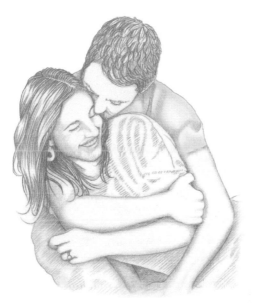

Do I need to use some sort of birth control right after delivery?

Before you resume intercourse be sure you have obtained an effective method of birth control. Birth control is necessary as you can become pregnant within the first few weeks after giving birth. Please refer to the section on "Family Planning Methods" (page 84).

You cannot rely on breast-feeding or the lack of menstruation to protect you against conceiving

Will intercourse be painful after delivery?

Communication about initial postpartum intercourse is as important as it was during pregnancy. Your tissues may still be tender and won't be as lubricated as they were before – so going slowly, talking with each other about what feels good and use of a water-soluble lubricant like K-Y jelly may be needed. Don't be discouraged if intercourse is uncomfortable or even a little painful. Your body needs to finish adjusting to a non-pregnancy state.

Postpartum Exercise Program

To help regain your figure and muscle tone, we recommend the following exercise program. If you start this program as soon as you get home from the hospital, be certain to start slowly. Avoid pushing yourself beyond the point that it hurts. If you notice any discomfort in the pelvis or any persistent changes in the vaginal discharge (such as color, odor, increased amount), stop the exercises and discuss these changes with your OB provider.

We recommend doing exercises 1 through 4 the first week. Add exercises 5 and 6 the second week. Exercises 7 and 8 can be added the third week. Each exercise should be repeated four times, twice a day.

First Week

Abdominal Breathing - Breathe in deeply to expand abdomen. Exhale slowly while drawing in abdominal muscles tightly.

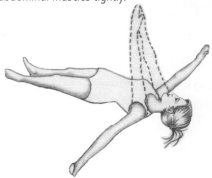

Arm Raising - Lie flat on floor, legs slightly apart. Stretch arms away from shoulders on floor with elbows stiff. Raise arms, elbows stiff, above torso and touch hands. Slowly return to the floor.

Neck Stretch - Lie flat on back, no pillows. Exhale and raise head to touch chin to chest.

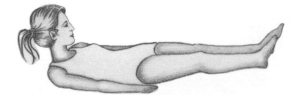

Kegel - This is the same exercise you did while pregnant to strengthen and control the muscles around the vagina (page 26). Tighten the muscles from front to the back (rectum) "like an elevator going up to the tenth floor," and then release very slowly one "floor" at a time.

Second Week

Pelvic Tilt - Lie on floor with knees bent. Inhale. While exhaling, flatten back hard against floor so that there is no space between back and floor. Tighten abdominal and buttock muscles as you flatten back.

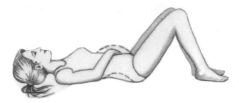

Knee Reach - Lie on your back with feet flat on floor, knees bent slightly. Lift your head and reach for (but don't touch) your left knee with your right hand. Repeat, using your right knee and left hand.

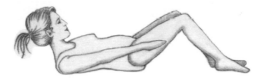

Third Week

Leg Raising - Lie flat on floor. Point toes. As you exhale, slowly raise leg to 45 degree angle. Inhale and lower leg slowly. Raise other leg. Repeat.

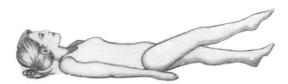

Modified Sit-Up - Lie back on floor, cross arms on chest, knees bent. Exhale and rise head and shoulders as you draw abdomen in. Inhale and slowly return to lying flat on the floor. (Do not do a "full sit-up.")

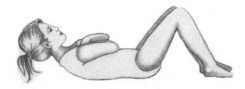

Family Planning Methods

Women seeking birth control have many different methods from which to choose. Family planning can be very important to your health. While individual needs vary greatly, if you and your partner decide to use birth control, you need a method that is effective, safe and easy for you to use.

There are many methods of birth control. The best one for you is the one that makes you feel comfortable and is suitable for your health and lifestyle. No matter which method you choose, no method will work unless you remember to use it, and do so correctly. Of sexually active women using no method of birth control, 90-100% will become pregnant in one year. Remember, breast-feeding and lack of menstruation are not methods of birth control.

Birth Control Pills/Contraceptive Patches/ Monthly Injections

How They Work: Pills/Patches/Injections are composed of two synthetic hormones, estrogen and progesterone. The contraceptive patch was approved in 2001. These methods prevent the release of an egg from the ovary and change the consistency of the cervical mucus so the sperm cannot reach the egg.

Advantages: Pills/Patches/Injections are 98-99% effective when used as directed. There are several advantages to taking hormones. They decrease the amount of monthly flow and anemia, decrease cramps in most patients, reduce occurrence of ovarian cysts, periods are more regular, help resolve acne and protect the lining of the uterus against cancer. Contraceptive patches are applied to the skin once weekly for 3 weeks. Injections are given at your doctor's office once a month. Some women find these methods easier than taking a pill daily.

Disadvantages: Pills/Patches/Injections have common side effects. These include nausea (usually limited to the first three months), changes in skin pigmentation, spotting between periods (usually clears within three months), and breast tenderness. Neither the pills, patches or injections protect against sexually transmitted diseases. Some women find injections uncomfortable.

You should not use birth control pills, Contraceptive patches or Monthly Injections if you:
- are 35 years or older and smoke.
- have a history of blood clots in legs or lungs or have had a heart attack.
- have a history of liver disease, high blood pressure or diabetes.
- take other medication that cannot be used along with birth control pills (check with your provider).
- think you might be pregnant.

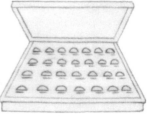

Note: Birth control pills (mini-pills) are available with only the progestin hormone (no estrogen) and can be used while breast-feeding (check with your provider).

Condoms - Female

How They Work: This is a female form of the male condom. It is made of latex and fits into the vagina of the woman before having intercourse. It is inserted similarly as the diaphragm and helps protect the woman against pregnancy and sexually transmitted diseases including AIDS (HIV infection), if used properly.

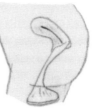

Advantages: Similar to the male condom.

Disadvantages: Takes practice to put in correctly. May decrease sensitivity during intercourse. Couple must be motivated to use each time they have intercourse.

Condoms - Male

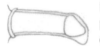

How They Work: The thin rubber covering is placed over the erect penis prior to intercourse to catch the semen and prevent it from entering the vagina.

Advantages: Can be bought over the counter. No harmful side effects. It is approximately 85-97% effective. Easy to use. Insertion can be incorporated as part of love making. Provides protection against venereal disease and common vaginal infections.

Disadvantages: Must be removed immediately after ejaculation to prevent slipping off when erection subsides. May break or slip off during vigorous intercourse. May cut down sensitivity. Occasional local allergic reaction. Couple must be motivated to use each time they have intercourse.

Contraceptive Injections (Depo-Provera)

How They Work: Contraceptive injections are an injectable form of a chemical similar to natural progesterone. This hormone prevents eggs, released from the ovaries, from ripening. If the egg is not ripe, it will not be released from the ovary and cannot be fertilized by sperm. This hormone also causes changes in the lining of the uterus that make it less likely for pregnancy to occur.

Advantages: Contraceptive injections are 99% affective if received every 3 months. Contraceptive injections are very convenient because there is nothing to remember to do daily, it cannot be expelled from your body and it is reversible. Most women who want to get pregnant, do so within 12-18 months after the last injection. Contraceptive injections can also be used while breast-feeding.

Disadvantages: Contraceptive injections must be given every 3 months (12 weeks) or you will not be protected against pregnancy. The major disadvantage of this method is irregular periods, especially in the first few months. Some women will also experience: weight gain, headaches, nervousness, stomach pain, dizziness, weakness, fatigue and lower sex drive. These injections do not protect you against sexually transmitted diseases.

Contraceptive Injections (Depo-Provera) Continued
You should not use Contraceptive injections if you:

- think you are pregnant.
- have had a stroke.
- have had liver disease.
- have had vaginal bleeding without knowing the cause.

- have had cancer of the breast.
- have had blood clots in your legs.
- are allergic to contraceptive injections.

Diaphragm

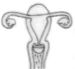

How They Work: The diaphragm covers the cervix, which is the opening into the uterus. The cover acts as a barrier to prevent the sperm from entering the uterus and the spermicide kills the sperm.

Advantages: The diaphragm is 94% effective, depending on whether it is used correctly and consistently. It is inexpensive and you don't have to remember to take medication. It can be inserted prior to love making or incorporated into love making. The diaphragm has been shown to decrease sexually transmitted diseases.

Disadvantages: It is only effective if used continuously and correctly. It must be left in place 6-8 hours after intercourse. On removal, it must be washed, dried, powdered and stored. Diaphragms must be fitted by a provider and replaced annually.

Non-surgical Permanent Birth Control
How They Work: Soft, flexible coils called "micro-inserts" are placed into each fallopian tube. These micro-inserts do not contain hormones. It takes 3 months for your body and the micro-inserts to form a tissue barrier to prevent pregnancy. A type of X-ray called a hysterosalpingogram (HSG) will be done at that time to make sure your tubes are completely blocked.

Advantages: No effect on hormones, menstruation, or sexual activity. This method is 99.8% effective. No cutting into your body. Rapid recovery - most women return to normal activities within 1 to 2 days. No general anesthesia.

Disadvantages: Procedure should be considered permanent and non-reversible. Must use a form of birth control for 3 months until HSG shows your tubes are completely blocked.

Foam, Cream, Jelly and Suppositories
How They Work: Inserted into the vagina before intercourse, they block the entrance to the uterus and the chemical content immobilize the sperm.

Advantages: Can be bought over the counter. No harmful side effects. Easy to use. Insertion can be incorporated as part of lovemaking and it is approximately 80-95% effective. When foam and condoms are used together, they are almost 99% effective.

Disadvantages: Suppositories require time to dissolve and may produce sensation of heat. Tend to be messy. Couple must be motivated to use each time they have intercourse. Occasional local allergic reaction.

Intrauterine Contraceptive (IUC/IUD)

There are two types of intrauterine contraceptives: the non-hormonal copper IUC and the hormonal IUC (Intrauterine System-IUS).

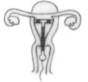

How They Work: The exact way an IUC works is not completely understood. They affect the mobility of the sperm, the egg, actual fertilization or implantation. The IUS, approved by the Food and Drug Administration in 2000, works the same way as the other IUC while using one hormone (progesterone) contained in oral contraceptives to prevent the release of an egg from the ovary. The IUS does not have the estrogen contained in some oral contraceptives, therefore avoiding the side effects associated with estrogen.

Advantages: The IUC is approximately 98-99% effective. The IUC is convenient and allows for complete spontaneity in sexual intercourse without having to take something every day. The IUC can be removed when a pregnancy is desired. It is recommended that the IUC strings be felt monthly. Women using the hormonal IUC may have lighter or no periods.

Disadvantages: Risk of pelvic infection is increased in the first 21 days after insertion. After the first 21 days the risk of infection is the same as a women without an IUC. Some women using the copper IUC have heavier periods or more cramping. Women with the hormonal IUC may have spotting between their periods.

IUCs are not recommended for:
• Women who think they might be pregnant
• Women with history of Pelvic Inflammatory Disease or sexually transmitted disease such as Gonorrhea or Chlamydia within 3 months before insertion

IUSs are not recommended for:
• Women with history of sexually transmitted disease similar to the IUC recommendations
• Women who think they might be pregnant
• Women who have had vaginal bleeding without knowing the cause, liver disease or breast cancer

Natural Family Planning

How They Work: Abstinence during ovulation when the woman is the most fertile. Involves observation of cervical mucus, basal body temperature and menstrual cycle.

Advantages: No drugs or devices needed. No physical side effects. Involves couple closely working together to make it 65-86% effective.

Disadvantages: Requires proper instructions, record keeping, observations and interpretations to be used effectively. Couple must abstain from intercourse on fertile days. Illness, infections and fever influence the observations.

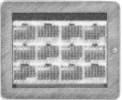

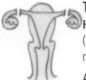

Tubal Coagulation or Ligation for Women

How They Work: The fallopian tubes are cut and tied or burned (coagulated) by an electric current so the egg cannot get through to meet the sperm.

Advantages: No effect on hormones, menstruation, or sexual activity. Freedom from fear of pregnancy and from use of temporary methods. This method is 99% effective.

Disadvantages: Procedure should be considered permanent and nonreversible in most cases. As with all surgery, there are risks of anesthesia complications, infection and bleeding.

Vaginal Ring

How They Work: This flexible plastic ring, approved by the Food and Drug Administration in 2001, contains estrogen and progesterone, similar to oral contraceptives (see "Oral Contraceptives," page 84) but in smaller amounts. The ring prevents the release of an egg from the ovary. The woman inserts this ring into the vagina for 3 weeks out of every month. A new ring must be used monthly.

Advantages: Vaginal rings are 98% effective when used as directed. One ring is inserted into the vagina every month and removed for 1 week for menses. Allows for spontaneity in love making without having to use a device or remembering to take a pill. Usually the sexual partner is unable to feel the ring during intercourse. Ring can be removed for up to 3 hours.

Disadvantages: Some women are not comfortable with the idea of inserting the ring vaginally. The woman needs to learn how to insert and remove the ring. Women may experience increased vaginal discharge.

You should not use the vaginal ring if you:
• think you might be pregnant.
• are 35 years or older and smoke.
• have a history of blood clots in legs or lungs or have had a heart attack.
• have a history of liver disease, high blood pressure or diabetes.
• take other medications that cannot be used along with hormones.

Vasectomy for Men

How They Work: The vas deferens tubes are cut and tied so the sperm does not get into the semen. The sperm is absorbed by the body.

Advantages: As with the tubal procedure for women, it is 99% effective. A minor procedure performed in the office under local anesthesia.

Disadvantages: Procedure is permanent and nonreversible in most cases. As with all surgery, there are risks of infection and bleeding. A temporary method of birth control must be used until there is a negative sperm count.

Post Delivery Check-up

Your first checkup will be scheduled approximately 5 to 6 weeks after delivery. The post delivery checkup will include the following:

- Blood pressure is checked to make sure that you do not have high blood pressure. Usually, blood pressure goes back to normal even if it was high during pregnancy. After pregnancy there is no longer a need for the extra blood your body produced to help nourish the baby and the placenta.

- A blood test may be done to make sure you are not anemic.

- Breast examination to check for any breast lumps and any nipple problems. If you are breast-feeding, your breasts may feel lumpy. Ask to be taught how to examine your own breasts.

- Vagina and cervix will be checked for abnormal bleeding, healing and muscle tone. A Pap smear may be done.

- Examination of the uterus for its size and shape. By 6 weeks postpartum, the uterus should be much smaller and the muscle walls thick and firm. The uterus never becomes quite as small as it was before you became pregnant.

- Abdominal check to assess your muscle tone.

- Advice on a birth control method and planning for the spacing of your future children should be discussed. You can get pregnant the first time you ovulate, which may be before you have a period. The first menstrual period can occur anywhere from 4 to 8 weeks (longer if breast-feeding) after delivery and the flow may be heavier than usual.

- Discussion about your feelings on being a new mother and the changes in your relationships with others.

"Postpartum blues" is no joke. If you find yourself depressed or unable to cope with your changed life after the baby is born, discuss your concerns with your OB provider and get some outside help right away.

Postpartum Questions

The postpartum checkup is a good time to ask any questions you may have about exercise, work, your health, your baby's health or anything else you do not understand or are concerned about.

Breast-Feeding

Breast-Feeding

A healthy mother can produce milk that is perfectly suited to her baby's needs. The American Academy of Pediatrics, the World Health Organization and the Surgeon General recommend breast-feeding. While exact amounts of protein, carbohydrates and fat in breast milk may vary from day-to-day, it will be right for your baby.

The reason that some women have trouble breast-feeding is possibly the lack of confidence, or not knowing some basic facts about breast-feeding. Obtaining accurate information on breast-feeding will help you gain confidence. Knowing how to solve problems you may encounter, such as inverted nipples, size and/or shape of your breasts, will help nursing go more smoothly.

Breast Changes During Pregnancy

While pregnant, your breasts are preparing to make milk for your baby. Milk is produced in sacs inside the breast. These sacs grow larger during pregnancy, and this causes your breasts to feel fuller, heavier and firmer. The area around the nipples, the areola, also becomes darker and perhaps larger. Small pimple-like glands (Montgomery's glands) may appear on areola.

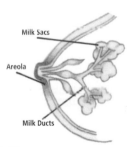

The size and shape of your breasts have nothing to do with successful breast-feeding.

Later in pregnancy, you may notice some colostrum, a yellow milk-like fluid, leaking from your nipples. This is normal, but it is also normal to have no leakage.

Bras for Pregnancy and Breast-Feeding

Studies have shown that there is no major change in breast size from nursing. Sagging breasts are not caused by nursing your baby, but by not wearing proper support while you are pregnant and nursing.

Nursing bras have special cups that open in the front to make it easier to feed. Your bra should be bought in the last months of pregnancy. Do not buy a bra with plastic liners in the cups, as these retain moisture and can contribute to infection. If you really like a bra but it happens to have plastic liners; you can cut them out before wearing it. It is good to purchase a bra "extender" at a notions counter as you may need the extra size as your milk first comes in.

Before buying your nursing bras, try on several and experiment fastening and unfastening the breast flap with one hand. This will help you find bras that not only work, but are also easy to use.

Preparation of the Breasts

Many practices have evolved to help prevent nipple soreness. Some of these practices have been studied for effectiveness and have proven ineffective, possibly even harmful to the pregnancy.

- Nipple rolling: designed to help pull the nipple erect, has been shown to cause premature labor, tetonic (very hard) contractions, and have not been shown to decrease soreness when breast-feeding.

- Buffing or rubbing with a towel: to "toughen" nipples can damage sensitive skin and does not decrease soreness. May also bring on contractions.

- Breast massage: designed to keep milk ducts open and prevent engorgement. It has not been proven to do either. However, massage of a particular duct (hard gland) when breast-feeding may help relieve a plugged duct.

- You may choose to use a nipple cream. There is some question as to whether it prevents soreness or if it heals soreness while breast-feeding.

What we suggest is that you become familiar with your breasts and the changes that are occurring. Continue your monthly breast exams and notice the differences in normal glandular increases. Remember to always clean your hands before handling the breasts.

Remember:

- Clean your breasts. Use a washcloth and water in your daily bath/shower. Soap should not be used as it dries out the natural oils.

- Wear a clean bra daily. Breast pads may be used if leaking occurs either before or after the baby is born. Change pads frequently and do not use plastic liners.

Colostrum

If you have not already noticed colostrum, or "first milk," coming from your breast before delivery, you will notice it soon after delivery. It is a special fluid that adequately feeds your baby for the first few days. It helps your baby to be immune to some illnesses, gives protection against diseases, infections and allergies. It is rich in protein. It also acts as a laxative, which helps your baby have bowel movements and helps prevent jaundice (the yellowing of the baby's skin). There is not as much quantity of this fluid as there will be of milk, but it is enough and good for your baby.

Milk Production

Milk production begins in response to hormones that are released upon the delivery of the placenta. These hormones are stimulated more by the baby's suckling. Relaxation is very important, as the mother who is tense can actually hold back hormone flow and thus decrease her milk flow. Be sure to breast-feed in a relaxed environment, alone or with those around with whom you are comfortable.

Although relaxation is very important in milk production, rest and good nutrition are also important. Rest and relax whenever you can the first week; fatigue can reduce your milk supply.

Factors Affecting Milk Supply

Your diet directly affects the quantity of your milk. You need the same well balanced meals you needed during pregnancy. Increase your protein and carbohydrate intake for an extra 500 calories a day. Drink plenty of liquids, as they are also important in milk production. You should drink approximately 10 to 12 8-ounce glasses of fluid daily. Review your suggested diet for breast-feeding earlier in this book in "Nutrition During Pregnancy," page 8.

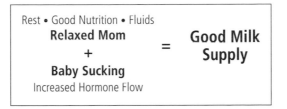

Rest • Good Nutrition • Fluids
Relaxed Mom
+
Baby Sucking
Increased Hormone Flow

= **Good Milk Supply**

Off To A Good Start

Proper placement is the key to a comfortable and successful breast-feeding experience. Begin by washing your hands before nursing your baby and getting into a comfortable position. If using the cradle hold (see Fig. 1), place a pillow on your lap to support baby

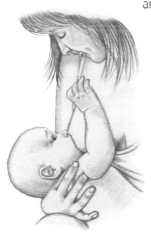

and another under the arm that holds baby and behind your back. If you are sitting in bed, bend your knees. If sitting in a chair, you will be more comfortable if you put your feet on a stool or extended out on another chair. Unwrap your baby if he is sleepy to stimulate him. Place him on his side, so that his lower arm goes around your midriff and the front of his body is facing the front of yours. He should be directly in front of your nipples. Baby's head should be in the bend of your elbow. (Fig. 1) With your free hand, place all fingers under your breast far enough back so that no fingers touch the areola (dark area around your nipple), with your thumb on top (see Fig. 2).

The "cigarette hold" (Fig. 3) prevents baby from latching on properly.

Fig. 1

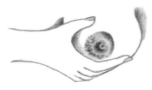

Fig. 2
Right Way

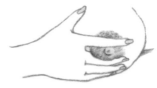

Fig. 3
Wrong Way

Gently tickle baby's lower lip with your nipple. This signals baby to open wide. BE PATIENT! When baby's mouth is very wide, quickly bring him close so his nose touches the breast (Fig. 4). Try to get as much of the areola (brown area surrounding the nipple) into the baby's mouth as possible. This way the baby can efficiently receive the breast milk. To give your baby adequate airway, pull his bottom closer. LISTEN! You will hear baby breathing. DO NOT press in with your thumb. Pressing in with your thumb will turn the nipple upward, causing a friction blister on the top of the nipple.

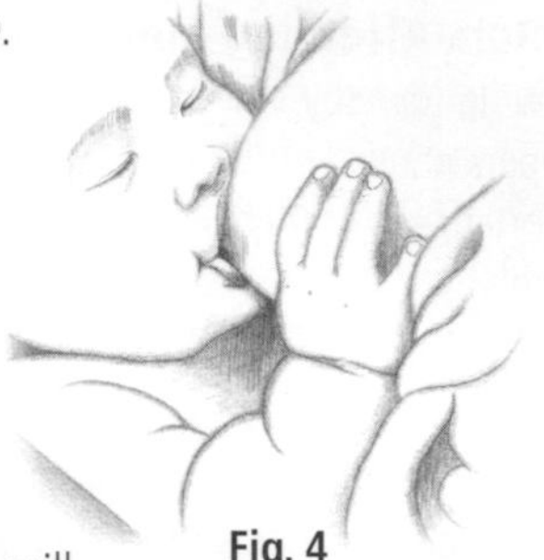

Fig. 4

You can feel the nipple being pulled out but there should not be pain. If it burns or "cuts" when baby sucks, put your finger in the corners of his mouth between his gums to break the suction and remove the baby from your breast. Then try again. Do not be discouraged. Many new mothers will have to try 5 to 10 times to get baby on correctly. If pain continues, ask for help in positioning. Do not wait until your nipples are cracked to ask for help.

How Long to Nurse

Watch your baby to give you clues as to how long to nurse. Most newborns will begin to slow down and doze off about 10 minutes into a feeding. That's the time to use your finger to break the suction and remove baby from your breast.

Now you can position yourself and baby to take the other breast and nurse until baby is satisfied and falls asleep. ALWAYS use your finger in baby's mouth when removing him from the breast to prevent him from biting down on the nipple again.

How Frequently To Nurse

As your baby grows older, more time will be spent in feeding, but feedings will be further apart. Since breast milk digests so easily, breast-fed newborns need to nurse every 1½ to 3 hours (8-12 times in 24 hours) around the clock. For this reason, you may wish to nurse lying down at night. Use the same positioning principles.

Leaking From Breasts

When baby nurses from one side, you may notice leaking from the other side. This is a good sign that your milk supply is in. Mature breast milk is very pale, almost bluish in color. This is normal and will provide proper nourishment for your baby. You may also notice leaking as you approach a feeding time or hear your baby cry. These are signs of the "letdown," but are not the only signs. Listen to baby as he suckles. If you hear him swallow (like sighs), you will know your milk is letting down adequately.

Is Baby Getting Enough?

How do you judge if your baby is getting enough? Your baby should have at least 8 wet diapers each day (some diapers are super absorbent and you may not change the baby as often) and 1 stool (bowel movement). The stools will go from black to green to yellow in color in the first weeks of life. Your pediatric provider will monitor your baby's weight gains.

Remember, all babies cry and sucking is their only means of calming themselves. If you just fed baby and he wakes as you put him down and begins sucking motions, he probably is not hungry. He may be frightened, lonely, cold, wet, positioned wrong or need wrapping with a blanket. If you wish to use a pacifier, discuss with your pediatric provider which is best to use.

Trouble Shooting

Engorgement: This may occur if nursing time is limited. You can relieve this fullness by nursing more frequently. Use warm cloths on breasts just prior to feeding. You may use acetaminophen (Tylenol) if needed, as prescribed by your OB provider. Massage while nursing may help empty the glands

If your breasts are very full, hand expression may be necessary to soften the areola enough for your baby to latch on. Do not pump breasts to empty them; you want the baby's nursing to regulate the amount of milk produced.

Sore nipples: Most of this can be prevented by proper placement of baby at the breast. If the nipples are sore as baby sucks, remove baby and reposition. Do not pull or push the top of your breast away from the baby's nose. This will cause the breast to be pulled from baby's mouth and he will only have to suck harder, creating blisters on the nipple. If you feel the baby can't breathe pull the baby's bottom in closer to you. Alternate the side you begin nursing on each feeding, using the least sore side first. Seek help before your nipples are damaged.

Allow breasts to air dry completely (10-15 minutes) after each feeding.

Breast pads and bras without plastic or polyester are necessary to protect nipples. Break suction before removing baby from your breast.

After nursing, allow a couple of drops of milk to drip on the nipples and rub on the nipple area. Then allow to air dry for 10-15 minutes.

If your baby is ever treated for thrush (yeast infection in the baby's mouth), you should also treat your breasts or the infection could pass back and forth from your baby to you.

Breast Infections - Mastitis

Sometimes a gland may not drain completely. You may notice hardness, generally near the underarm. You can begin using heat and massage in an effort to relieve this. If, however, redness, pain or a fever occurs, an infection may be present. See your OB provider for treatment. In most cases you may continue to breast-feed your baby.

Expressing Milk

You may at some time find it necessary to express milk from your breasts. This may be because you wish to have a bottle of breast milk for a future feeding, or you may be away from baby for some reason and need to empty your breasts. Milk you have expressed from your breast is good for only 48 hours if stored in your refrigerator. It may be kept in the back of your freezer section for up to 8 weeks. Never express milk and put into a bottle with milk from another time of expression. Label all bottles with date that you expressed.

Manually Express Milk

• Wash your hands. Use a sterilized glass or plastic bottle.

• Place the thumb on the tip of the breast just behind the areola and all fingers on the bottom of the breast just behind the areola. Support the breast by lifting it up (Fig. 1).

• Gently push together with thumb and fingers while pushing toward chest wall. Do not pull out as if "milking a cow" (Fig. 2).

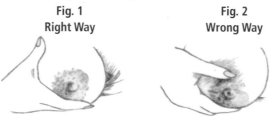

Fig. 1
Right Way

Fig. 2
Wrong Way

• Rotate the thumb and fingers around the areola, pushing back in each area. This will compress each of the storage ducts.

• A funnel that is attached to the bottle may make hand-expressed milk easier to collect. A wide mouth measuring cup or flexible plastic bowl may also be used and makes pouring into a bottle easier.

Use Pump to Express Milk

• Wash your hands. Be sure pump has been cleaned well.

• Place opening of pump on the breast, making sure a tight seal is obtained.

• Follow manufacturer's instructions for the pump you have purchased.

• Wash the pump with soap and water, rinsing it well.

• Remember you will never get as much with a pump as baby gets when nursing.

If you need milk for a future feeding, pump midway between two feedings. You may have to do this between several feedings to collect enough for one feeding. Be sure to use a separate bottle each time.

If you are not getting enough rest at night during the first few months, you may want to have someone else give the baby a night feeding. A bottle of formula or earlier pumped breast milk can be given occasionally, as you do need rest to keep up your milk supply. This should be done infrequently or your milk supply will decrease. The more you formula-feed your baby, the less milk you will make. To avoid confusing the baby about breast and bottle-feeding, it is better to introduce a bottle only after breast-feeding is well established, usually 3-4 weeks.

Nursing Privately In Public

You will find breast-feeding in public more comfortable if you:

- wear two-piece outfits rather than dresses. Shirts or blouses that can be pulled up from the waist allows the baby to nurse and his head covers any exposed area. If your blouse buttons down the front, unbutton it from the bottom rather than the top. "Nursing tops" are also available in some stores.

- wear light colors and patterned fabrics the first two weeks, as they will show less wetness if you should leak occasionally.

- put a hat on the baby as this gives more covering of any exposed areas of the breast. Sometimes it is more difficult to start and finish breast-feeding without attracting attention than the actual breast-feeding. You may want to start a feeding in private and then join family members or friends.

Nursing in public becomes more comfortable with practice.

Wearing loose-fitting clothes; covering your nursing baby with a diaper or receiving blanket is also good camouflage.

An easy place to nurse is the dressing room of department stores. In restaurants, booths are better for nursing than a table. Your parked car is also a good place to breast-feed if the weather permits. You can almost always find a good place to nurse, but try not to use the restroom unless the restroom has a separate lounge with chairs. A bathroom certainly is not a very pleasant place for a meal.

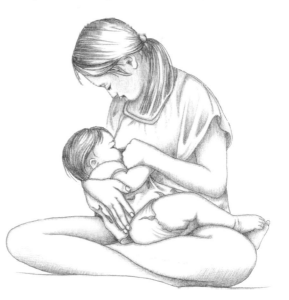

Practice at home before going outside, and you will have an easy transition to nursing privately in public.

Glossary

AFP (Alpha Feto Protein): Fetal (baby) protein that can be measured in the mother's blood.

Afterbirth: The placenta and membranes that pass out of the uterus during the third stage of labor.

Afterpains (af ter-pains): The cramping discomfort due to contractions of the uterus that is felt by some women after the birth of a child.

Amniocentesis (am -ne-o-sen-te -sis): A needle is inserted through the mother's abdomen (stomach) into the amniotic sac to withdraw fluid for examination.

Amniotic Fluid (am-ni-ot ic): Water-like fluid contained in the membranous sac surrounding the baby that serves to help support the baby, to permit movement of the baby, to prevent loss of heat and to absorb shocks.

Amniotic Sac (am-ni-ot ic): Membrane or tissue that surrounds the baby and is filled with amniotic fluid. Sometimes called "bag of waters."

Anemia (ah-ne -me-ah): A deficiency in the blood, either in quality or quantity.

Antepartum: The period of pregnancy from conception to delivery.

Antibody (an -ti -bod -e): A protein that is produced in the body in response to an invasion by a foreign agent.

Areola (a-re o-lah): The pigmented rings surrounding the nipple of the breast.

Bladder: Organ that collects and stores urine.

Braxton-Hick's Contractions: (see False Labor).

Breech: The buttock; delivery of the baby with buttocks or legs first.

Catheter (kath -e-ter): A small rubber tube used to drain urine from the bladder.

Centimeters: The unit of measurement used to describe progress in dilation; used interchangeably with "fingers," - one "finger" equaling two centimeters.

Cervical os (ser vi-cal oss): The ordinarily small opening of the cervix that dilates during the first stage of labor.

Cervix (ser vix): Narrow end of the uterus, opening into the vagina.

Chromosomes (kro mo soms): Present in all cells of the body, contain genes or hereditary factors that are passed on to the fetus by its parents.

Complete: A term used to indicate complete dilation of the cervix. A woman is said to be "complete" when the cervix is sufficiently dilated for the baby to pass through, usually ten centimeters or five "fingers". In terms of inches, the completely dilated cervix usually measures about four inches in diameter or 13 1/2 inches in circumference.

Conception: The union of sperm and egg resulting in new life; fertilization.

Contractions: Tightening and shortening of the uterine muscles during labor causing effacement (thinning) and dilation (opening) of the cervix and contributing to the downward and outward passage of the baby; sometimes called "pains."

Crowning: Appearance of the presenting part of the baby at the perineum during the second stage of labor.

Dilation (dil a-tion): The gradual opening and drawing up of the cervix to permit passage of the baby.

Doppler: An instrument that utilizes sound waves in order to hear the baby's heart beat.

EDC (Estimated Day of Confinement): The date that is calculated to be the date of delivery (280 days or 40 weeks).

Edema (ĕ-de mah): Abnormal accumulation of fluids in the intercellular spaces of the body (face, hands, legs and feet).

Effacement (ef-face ment): Thinning of the cervix.

Embryo (em bree-o): The scientific term for the baby during the second through the eighth week in the uterus.

Engagement: Process whereby the presenting part of the baby secures itself into the upper opening (inlet) of the pelvic canal and is in its beginning position for passage through this circular, bony structure. May be noticed by the mother as "lightening," usually occurring two weeks before onset of labor.

Engorgement: Fullness of the breasts due to milk production. Experienced by both nursing and non-nursing mothers.

Epidural (ep ĭ-du ral): A type of anesthesia used during labor and delivery. A small tube is placed into the epidural space of the spine and pain medication is administered.

Episiotomy (e-pi zi-ot o-mee): An incision made into the perineum prior to delivery for the purpose of preventing tears and facilitating delivery.

Fallopian Tubes (fah-lo pe-an): The two small tubes extending from either side of the uterus toward the left and right ovary. When the ripened egg is expressed from the ovary, it is received into the fallopian tube.

False Labor (Braxton-Hick's Contractions): Regular and irregular contractions of the uterus may be painless or strong enough to be interpreted as true labor but that have no dilating effect on the cervix.

Fertilization: Fusion of the sperm and egg normally occurring in the fallopian tubes; conception.

Fetal Alcohol Syndrome: The results seen in some babies when the mother consumes alcohol while she is pregnant.

Fetal Heart Tones (FHT): The baby's heartbeat as heard with an instrument through the mother's abdominal wall.

Fetus (feet us): The scientific term for the baby from the end of the third month of pregnancy until delivery.

Forceps (for-seps): Instruments occasionally used to assist delivery of the baby.

Fundus (fun dus): The upper portion of the uterus.

Gravid (gra vid): Pregnant.

Gestation: The condition or period of carrying a baby in the uterus.

Hematocrit (he-mat -o-krit): The volume percent of red blood cells in the blood.

Hemoglobin (he -mo-glo -bin): The oxygen carrying part of the blood.

Hyperventilation (hi -per-ven-ti-la shun): Abnormally prolonged and deep breathing, usually associated with acute anxiety or emotional tension.

Implantation: The attaching and embedding of a fertilized egg in the uterine lining.

Involution (in vo-lu tion): Return of the female reproductive organs (uterus) to their non-pregnant state after delivery, taking approximately six weeks.

Labia (la be-ah): External folds around opening of the vagina.

Lightening: Movement of the baby and the uterus downward into the pelvic cavity; "dropping;" engagement.

Lochia (lo kee-a): Discharge of blood, mucous, and tissue from the uterus after the birth of a baby, that may continue several weeks.

Mature Milk: That which comes in the breasts after the colostrum, 3-4 days after delivery.

Meconium (me-ko nee-um): The dark green or black substance present in the baby's large intestine at birth that he/she passes for the first few days.

Membranes: The membranous sac or bag that contains amniotic fluid. Also known as the "amniotic sac" or the "bag of waters."

Mucus Plug: A plug of heavy mucus that blocks the cervical canal during pregnancy.

Multipara (mul-tip ah-rah): A woman who has had a previous birth.

Nullipara (nu-lip ah-rah): A woman who has not yet given birth to a baby.

OB provider/Provider: The person that is responsible for a woman's medical care during her pregnancy (i.e., Doctor, Nurse Practitioner, Physician's Assistant).

Pelvis: The bony ring that joins the spine and legs. (Its central opening forms the walls of the birth canal.)

Perineum (per i-nee um): The tissue between the rectum and the vulva (vagina).

Placenta (pla-sen ta): The vascular structure developed in pregnancy through which nutrition and excretion take place between mother and baby; commonly known as the "afterbirth."

Placenta Previa: Placenta that is located on the lower part of the uterus and covers a part or all of the cervix.

Postpartum: After delivery.

Post-mature Pregnancy: A pregnancy that has gone past the calculated date of delivery, usually considered to be 41 to 42 weeks.

Prenatal: Before giving birth.

Pre-term Labor: Labor that occurs before the completion of the 37th week of pregnancy.

Primipara (pri-mip a-ra): A woman having her first baby.

Quickening: The first movements of the fetus felt by the mother; "feeling life."

Rh Factor: An additional blood factor that is present in 85% or more of the population. When it is absent, the person is said to be Rh negative.

Ripe: A term used to describe the condition of the cervix when ready for the onset of labor.

Second Stage of Labor: The period of time from full dilation (10 cm) of the cervix to when the baby passes from the uterus through the vagina and is born. This may take anywhere from a few minutes to several hours.

Show: The reddish-colored mucus, that sometimes announces the onset of labor or is gradually discharged during labor; the sloughing off of the protective mucus plug that seals over the cervix during pregnancy.

Sperm: Male reproductive cell.

Third Stage of Labor: The period of time after the baby is born until the time when the placenta is dislodged and expelled, lasting on the average from one to twenty minutes.

Transition: The end of the first stage of labor; the period of dilation from about eight to ten centimeters, usually lasting about 15 to 25 minutes.

Trimester (tri-mes ter): A period of three months.

Umbilical Cord (um-bil ĭ-kal): The cord connecting the umbilicus of the baby to the placenta.

Umbilicus (um-bil ĭ-kus): The navel or "belly button."

Urethra (u-re thrah): The tube that carries urine from the bladder to outside the body.

Uterus (u ter-us): The organ of gestation, consisting of a pear-shaped fundus and a narrower, lower portion called the cervix; the womb.

Varicose (var ĭ-kōs): Unnaturally dilated vein.

Vertex (ver tex): Top of the head; delivery of the baby with head first.

Vulva (vul vah): The external female reproductive organs; generally understood as the external lips or folds, that precede the vaginal entrance.

Index

About the Author

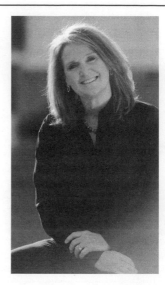

Kendis Moore Drake - Mother, RN, FNP and Olympian

When Kendis began caring for pregnant women 25 years ago, she tried to find a concise, easy-to-read book that would help educate her patients about their pregnancies. No such book existed, so Kendis wrote this book to help expectant mothers understand the wonderful process of pregnancy and delivery. Universities, doctors' offices, health plans, health departments, clinics and hospitals throughout the country have used *Preparing For A Healthy Baby* for more than 20 years. Now this book is available directly to expectant mothers.

Kendis graduated magna cum laude from Arizona State University with both her Bachelor's of Science degree and Master's degree in Nursing. Kendis is a former world record holder in swimming and Olympic team member. She continues to enjoy sports and caring for patients, while expanding her practice to include gynecology and women's health.